ACUTE CORONARY SYNDROME WITH COMORBIDITIES

A Therapeutic Challenge

ACUTE CORONARY SYNDROME WITH COMORBIDITIES

A Therapeutic Challenge

Author

Gurunath Parale MD DM FACC FCSI FICP
Professor
Department of Medicine
Ashwini Rural Medical College

Chief Cardiologist
Ashwini Cooperative Hospital
Solapur, Maharashtra, India

Editorial Assistance

Virupaksha Joshi MBBS DMRD
Radiologist
Ashwini Cooperative Hospital
Solapur, Maharashtra, India

Forewords

D Prabhakaran
George Joseph
Jagdish S Hiremath
CK Ponde

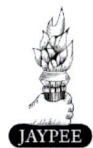

JAYPEE BROTHERS MEDICAL PUBLISHERS
The Health Sciences Publisher
New Delhi | London

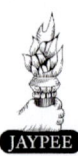 **Jaypee Brothers Medical Publishers (P) Ltd**

Headquarters
EMCA House
23/23-B, Ansari Road, Daryaganj
New Delhi 110 002, India
Landline: +91-11-23272143,
+91-11-23272703
+91-11-23282021, +91-11-23245672
E-mail: jaypee@jaypeebrothers.com

Corporate Office
Jaypee Brothers Medical Publishers (P) Ltd.
4838/24, Ansari Road, Daryaganj
New Delhi 110 002, India
Phone: +91-11-43574357
Fax: +91-11-43574314
E-mail: jaypee@jaypeebrothers.com

Overseas Office
JP Medical Ltd.
83, Victoria Street, London
SW1H 0HW (UK)
Phone: +44-20 3170 8910
E-mail: info@jpmedpub.com

EU GPSR Authorised Representative
Logos Europe, 9 rue Nicolas Poussin
17000, La Rochelle, France
Phone: +33 (0) 6 67 93 73 78
E-mail: Contact@logoseurope.eu

Website: www.jaypeebrothers.com
Website: www.jaypeedigital.com

© 2020, Jaypee Brothers Medical Publishers

The views and opinions expressed in this book are solely those of the original contributor(s)/author(s) and do not necessarily represent those of editor(s) of the book.

All rights reserved. No part of this publication may be reproduced, stored or transmitted in any form or by any means, electronic, mechanical, photocopying, recording or otherwise, without the prior permission in writing of the publishers.

All brand names and product names used in this book are trade names, service marks, trademarks or registered trademarks of their respective owners. The publisher is not associated with any product or vendor mentioned in this book.

Medical knowledge and practice change constantly. This book is designed to provide accurate, authoritative information about the subject matter in question. However, readers are advised to check the most current information available on procedures included and check information from the manufacturer of each product to be administered, to verify the recommended dose, formula, method and duration of administration, adverse effects and contraindications. It is the responsibility of the practitioner to take all appropriate safety precautions. Neither the publisher nor the author(s)/editor(s) assume any liability for any injury and/or damage to persons or property arising from or related to use of material in this book.

This book is sold on the understanding that the publisher is not engaged in providing professional medical services. If such advice or services are required, the services of a competent medical professional should be sought.

Every effort has been made where necessary to contact holders of copyright to obtain permission to reproduce copyright material. If any have been inadvertently overlooked, the publisher will be pleased to make the necessary arrangements at the first opportunity. The **CD/DVD-ROM** (if any) provided in the sealed envelope with this book is complimentary and free of cost. **Not meant for sale.**

Inquiries for bulk sales may be solicited at: jaypee@jaypeebrothers.com

Acute Coronary Syndrome with Comorbidities: A Therapeutic Challenge / Gurunath Parale

First Edition: 2020, Reprint: **2025**

ISBN: 978-93-89129-91-5

Printed in India

Dedication

I dedicate this book to my teachers at medical school who instilled in me, during those formative years, a sense of enquiry and inquisitiveness about everything. They gave me not just the fish, but also the fishing rod and moreover taught me how to use the rod.

ABOUT THE AUTHOR

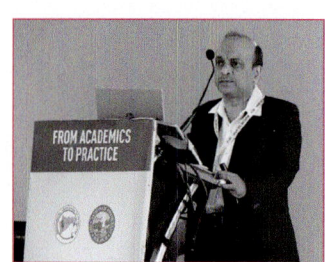

- DM Cardiology from PGIMER (Chandigarh)
- Trained in CMC (Vellore), CTC (Liverpool)
- Chief Cardiologist, Ashwini Hospital, Solapur
- Professor Medicine, Ashwini Rural Medical College, Solapur
- Fellow of American College of Cardiology
- More than 30,000 Angiographies/Angioplasties
- More than 300,000 Echocardiograms/Stress Tests
- More than 40 Publications in International and National Journals
- 122 Citations by Authors from all over the World
- Numerous Paper/Case Presentations/Lectures in India and Abroad including Prestigious Conferences like PCR in Paris, TCT in San Francisco, ESC in Rome
- Recipient of Rotary Millennium Award, *Sharad Puraskar*, Gandhi Forum Award
- Authored a Book '*Sahriday*' and VCD for Patient Education.

FOREWORD

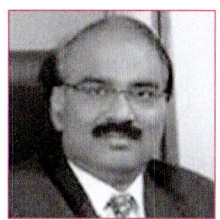

D Prabhakaran MD DM (Cardiology) MSc FRCP FNASc
Vice President - Research and Policy, Public Health Foundation of India (PHFI)

Professor, Department of Epidemiology
London School of Hygiene and Tropical Medicine, UK

Former Professor, Cardiology
All India Institute of Medical Sciences

Cardiovascular diseases have become the leading cause of death in India. According to the state level disease burden published recently they contribute nearly 20% of total mortality. Despite this they pose both a great challenge as well as an immense opportunity to healthcare providers in the world. While the survival has considerably improved, the biggest challenge in India is that the disease occurs at younger ages imposing an unaffordable financial burden to individuals and their families. In addition, comorbidities have emerged as a major determinant of survival among patients with coronary artery disease.

When I was asked to review the book titled "Acute Coronary Syndrome with Comorbidities: A Therapeutic Challenge" by the well-known cardiologist Dr Gurunath Parale from Solapur, Maharashtra. I wondered as to the need for another book of cardiology given the profusion of textbooks that are currently available. However, ongoing through the book in detail, I am sure that this book will find a unique niche both for students and practicing cardiologists. One of the most ignored aspects in the management of coronary artery diseases is the presence of comorbidities and there is hardly any patient without involvement of another organ system which substantially influences outcomes and increases mortality. Dr Parale has had years of experience in handling such comorbidities and has shared his experiences through case studies. This format provides a real-life scenario and many of us can easily relate to such situations. In addition, he has provided several practical tips in handling patients with comorbidities. Further, the simple English makes it easily readable and I am sure this book will become a ready reckoner for the practicing cardiologist in handling complex situations.

My hearty congratulations to Dr Parale in writing this book which must have been a love of labor for him. I am sure this book will be widely read and used.

FOREWORD

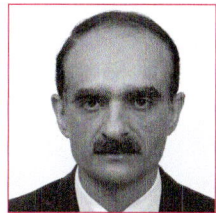

George Joseph DM FCSI
Professor of Cardiology
Christian Medical College
Vellore, Tamil Nadu, India

An outstanding masterpiece from a brilliant academician, this gem of a book is a must-read for any clinician dealing with coronary artery disease patients. Dr Gurunath Parale has a captivating style of presentation, starting each chapter by narrating related real-life dilemmas he encountered candidly and with endearing honesty. Having whetted the appetite to know more about the subject, Dr Parale then launches into a masterly review of the relevant literature, providing fascinating insights into the pathophysiology and management of acute coronary syndrome encountered in association with various comorbidities. The primary focus is on the practical difficulties one often faces when dealing with patients with acute coronary syndrome and specific comorbidities. Dr Parale provides clear solutions to each problem, based on a thorough but succinct review of the state-of-the-art and the latest guidelines. And if this was not enough to indelibly imprint these facts in one's memory, Dr Parale provides a deft finishing touch to each chapter with a precise summary of the key points. I am sure anyone fortunate enough to lay hands on a copy of this book will enjoy reading it as much as I did.

FOREWORD

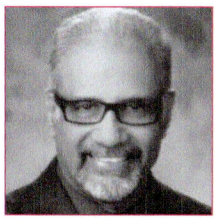

Jagdish S Hiremath DM (Card) DNB (Card) FACC
Director
Cath Lab Ruby Hall Clinic
Pune, Maharashtra, India

I have been associated with Dr Gurunath Parale as a professional colleague for many decades. His astute clinical judgement supported with exceptional hand skill makes him one of the leading interventional cardiologist of the country. Present book of comorbid conditions with acute coronary syndrome, the subject of the book itself indicates a thinker in Dr Gurunath Parale. The chapters that you will read are real-world experiences. Dr Parale always follows guideline science, but also adds original experience in the narration. He is a master of science of medicine, but also introduces art of medicines which comes from the book of experience.

I find this book exceptionally useful for all interventional cardiologists. It is an excellent reference book in one's shelf and in one's computer. Every chapter can guide one when faced with "associated comorbid conditions with acute coronary syndrome". I congratulate Dr Gurunath Parale for having thought of this unusual topic and passing the benefit of his own thought process to many of his colleagues like me and also thousands of junior budding cardiologist of the country.

FOREWORD

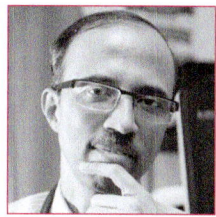

CK Ponde MBBS MD DM
Consultant Cardiologist
PD Hinduja National Hospital and Medical Research Centre
Mumbai, Maharashtra, India

It gives me great pleasure and pride to write a foreword for Dr Gurunath's venture. Postgraduate medicine is ever evolving and this is the era of evidence-based medicine. The textbook knowledge of the disease process forms the base of the pyramid and pyramid keeps on going taller when more and more data is added derived from randomized trials and registries. A clinician is supposed to have mandatory knowledge of clinical trials and registry data which help him in decision making in day-to-day clinical practice. Despite this knowledge, there are frequent occasions where a clinician is faced with a case where decision making is extremely difficult, complex and challenging.

I myself firmly believe that the use of clinical case discussions is one of the best method of teaching and learning medicine not only for the medical students, but also for experienced consultants.

Dr Gurunath Parale is known to the medical world for a very long time. He was the pioneer cardiologist in the district of Solapur and has practiced medicine and all the facets of cardiology including clinical cardiology, echocardiography and interventional cardiology in the most versatile manner. He has maintained his academic excellence even when having the busiest practice and that too in a place like Solapur. He has written books for patients, has published several articles in national and international journals and also has presented complex interventional cases in conferences like TCT and EuroPCR.

This compilation of challenging case scenarios and dilemmas in cardio-vascular medicine comes as a breath of fresh air. He has beautifully discussed each case/topic, its complexity in a most lucid manner with extensive coverage of the relevant literature. What is most important is that the clinicians will get a very clear idea about how to deal with such dilemma when they face such a patient. The selection of cases and the topics explore those areas of cardiology which remains untouched in textbooks, journals and even conferences.

I am extremely impressed with this book because it bridges the gap between the established knowledge and the gray areas and this is so very important for a clinical cardiologist today, because he/she is invariably faced with patients with multiple comorbidities.

I and Dr Gurunath have a very long association of over 30 years, as we both have taken our postgraduate degrees in medicine from the same institute, VM Medical College, Solapur, Maharashtra. When I look back and see his growth it makes me immensely proud and ecstatic.

At the end, I must say that if every clinician keeps on contributing such pearls of experience to help his colleagues and budding consultants the world will become a different place.

PREFACE

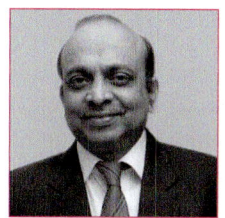

Gurunath Parale MD DM FACC FCSI FICP
Professor
Department of Medicine
Ashwini Rural Medical College
Chief Cardiologist
Ashwini Cooperative Hospital
Solapur, Maharashtra, India

It is almost 25 years since I embarked on my practice of cardiology in the 'textile town' of Solapur, Maharashtra, India. Since I was the only cardiologist with super-specialist qualification for a long time, it was not surprising that patients from all corners of this large district were referred to me for consultation on various heart ailments. The diagnosis and treatment of ischemic heart disease used to be a relatively simple affair with straight-forward approach as guided by the standard textbooks. Once the acute myocardial infarction (AMI) was diagnosed acute coronary syndrome (ACS) is a recent nomenclature, based on TMT and ECG findings, the treatment options were 2-fold, i.e. either intravenous thrombolysis, if the patient reached the hospital within the so-called 'window' period or a conservative line of management with bed-rest and medications. It was the era before the hi-tech cath labs and percutaneous re-perfusion techniques became the standard, first-line methods of treatment.

However, in the past decade or so, the scene of cardiology practice changed in significant ways. Firstly, I was no longer the only cardiologist and the hospital, where I worked was not the only hospital catering to the district inhabited by a million people. The so-called simple and uncomplicated cases of ACS were successfully treated in smaller nursing homes at the periphery of the district. Secondly, the not-so-simple cases were being referred to the tertiary care hospital where I work. Many of the patients referred to me with heart disease suffered from other comorbid conditions. Some of them had a long history of chronic obstructive airway disease, while some others had suffered a recent cerebrovascular accident. Many of these patients with heart disease had a hitherto undetected kidney disease or a hematological disorder or even a connective tissue disease. Some of the patients who were referred to me for cardiac evaluation were even treated and declared as cured from malignant disease such as breast carcinoma. At least two of the patients suffered from chronic liver disease and one of them was even wait-listed for a liver transplant. Therefore, the present scene was a far cry from the old days when I diagnosed AMI and treated it with thrombolysis or waited with crossed fingers for the patient to recover after prescribing medicines.

However, with the advent of primary angioplasty as the treatment of choice for AMI, a paradigm shift took place in the manner in which MI or ACS was treated. Introduction of drug-eluting stents was a path-breaking innovation and dual antiplatelet therapy became the mainstay of medication to prevent thrombosis within the stent. However, the changing demography of the patients referred to a tertiary care hospital had its own share of challenges. Apart from the cardiac disease, associated comorbid conditions in some of them threw up special challenge for the treating cardiologists like me. For instance:

- Could I go ahead with a PCI with a drug-eluting stent followed by heparin and dual antiplatelet therapy in a patient with advanced liver disease and GI bleed?
- Can I proceed with PCI and dual antiplatelet therapy in a patient with a recent intracerebral hematoma and risk further increase in the size of the hematoma and neurological deterioration?
- How safe it is to proceed with coronary angiography involving potentially nephrotoxic contrast media in a patient with pre-existing renal dysfunction?

These are some of the vexed issues troubling the cardiologist like me practicing in a tertiary care hospital. Moreover, there is scanty and sketchy material available in present day medical literature to guide the physician and help him practice evidence-based medicine. The book in your hand now is a culmination of my decade-long effort to find meaningful answers and dependable protocols to deal with the vexed problem of heart disease with comorbid conditions. It is my ardent hope that the reader will find answers in this book to the dilemma he/she must be facing in his/her daily practice.

ACKNOWLEDGMENTS

I am indebted to my wife *Dr Neha*, without whose moral support this book would not have been possible. Silently but stoically, *Dr Neha* put up with my obsession to write this book and the manner in which this obsession intruded our 'we' time even during weekends and holidays. I am grateful to my elder son *Dr Chinmay* for his insightful comments and suggestions. I discovered during these interactions what a fine young man he has turned out to be. I also acknowledge my younger son *Hrishikesh* whose encouraging words have kept me steadfast on my path toward academic pursuit.

I am honoured and obligated to well acclaimed quartet of cardiologists Dr D Prabhakaran, New Delhi, Dr George Joseph, Vellore, Dr Jagdish S Hiremath, Pune, Dr CK Ponde, Mumbai. Each one of them not only set aside his precious time to read excerpts of this book but also readily agreed to write a foreword. Without the encouraging forewords from such accomplished cardiologists and prominent academicians, this book would not have acquired the legitimacy I hope it would.

I also acknowledge *Dr Satyawan Sharma*, the famous cardiologist at Bombay Hospital who gave me some useful suggestions.

Last but not the least, important is the invaluable help I got from my colleague radiologist *Dr Virupaksha Joshi*. Although his specialty is far different from the topics in this book, he put his mind, brain and most importantly heart into this project and helped me to complete it which at one point of time I thought was not possible.

CONTENTS

1. Introduction — 1
2. Acute Coronary Syndrome with Stroke — 6
3. Acute Coronary Syndrome with Chronic Kidney Disease — 29
4. Acute Coronary Syndrome Patients needing Anticoagulation — 49
5. Acute Coronary Syndrome with Chronic Obstructive Pulmonary Disease — 58
6. Acute Coronary Syndrome with Chronic Liver Disease — 68
7. Acute Coronary Syndrome in Hematological Disorders — 81
8. Acute Coronary Syndrome in Cancer — 90
9. Acute Coronary Syndrome with Connective Tissue Diseases — 105
10. Acute Coronary Syndrome with Human Immunodeficiency Virus Infections — 116
11. Perioperative Myocardial Infarction — 122

Index — 129

CHAPTER 1

Introduction

Cardiovascular disease (CVD) is a dominant cause of sickness and death all over the world. It accounts for almost 30% of all-cause mortality in the world.[1] Since the burden of CVD increases with age, it is not surprising that a major portion of the patients with CVD tend to be older and frailer with multiple comorbidities. Presence of a comorbid condition not only affects the disease progression in CVD but also profoundly influences clinical outcome and decision-making. It is a known that cardiovascular comorbidities such as hypertension, diabetes, atrial fibrillation, heart failure and stroke are independent predictors of risk and mortality in patients presenting to the emergency department of a hospital with acute myocardial infarction (AMI). However, the fact that many of the patients with CVD harbor a broad spectrum of noncardiovascular comorbidities receives less attention. The cardiovascular and noncardiovascular morbidities such as chronic obstructive pulmonary disease (COPD), liver cirrhosis, chronic kidney disease (CKD) and connective tissue disorders have a significant bearing on presentation, management and prognosis of CVD (Figs. 1 and 2).[2]

The Charlson comorbidity index (CCI) is a well-recognized measure of comorbid conditions.[3] It quantifies prognostic impact of twenty-two comorbid conditions by means of a score—making it a useful tool for objective assessment of prognosis in multiple coexisting illnesses.

Different variables in Charlson comorbidity index with respective score are as follows:
- Cerebrovascular disease: 1
- Congestive heart failure: 1
- Peripheral vascular disease: 1
- Myocardial infarction: 1
- Connective tissue disease: 1
- Dementia: 1
- Chronic obstructive pulmonary disease: 1

- Peptic ulcer disease: 1
- Moderate-to-severe CKD: 2
- Leukemia: 2
- Hemiplegia: 2
- Malignant lymphoma: 2
- AIDS: 6
- Diabetes mellitus: 1 (if uncomplicated) and 2 (if end organ is damaged)
- Liver disease: 1 (if mild) and 2 (if moderate-to-severe)
- Solid tumor (any): 2
- Metastatic solid tumor: 6.

Many randomized controlled studies from a wide spectrum of populations have shown that majority of the patients with CVD have at least one comorbidity. Over the years, the prevalence of comorbidity has shown an upward trend. Conversely, the number of CVD patients without comorbidity has steadily fallen during the past couple of decades.

A meta-analysis by Rashid et al. looked at the impact of CCI on the outcomes in following cardiovascular conditions:
- Acute coronary syndrome (ACS)
- Stable coronary heart disease (CHD)
- Patients undergoing percutaneous intervention (PCI).

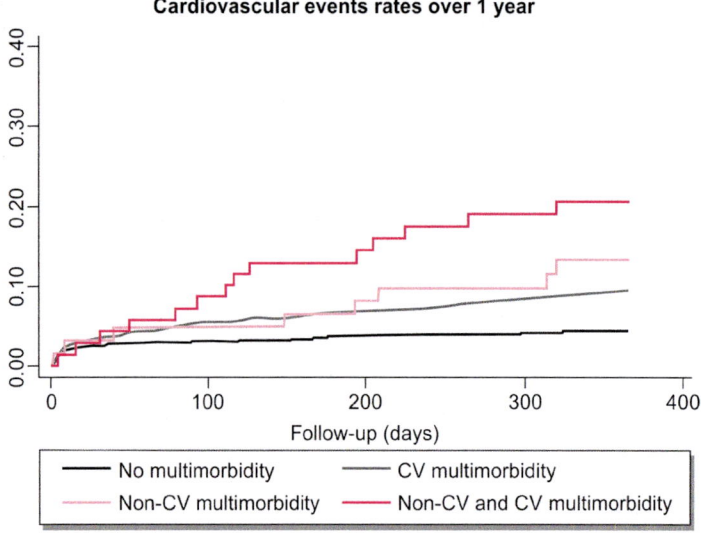

FIG. 1: Showing prognostic influence of cardiac and noncardiac comorbidities on cardiovascular events.

Source: Canivell S, Muller O, Gencer B, et al. Prognosis of cardiovascular and non-cardiovascular multimorbidity after acute coronary syndrome. PLoS One. 2018;13(4):e0195174.

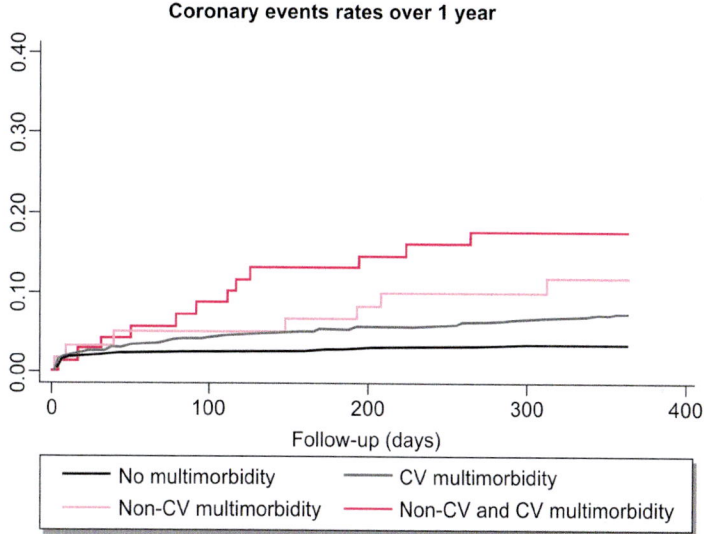

FIG. 2: Showing impact of cardiac and noncardiac comorbidities on coronary events.
Source: Canivell S, Muller O, Gencer B, et al. Prognosis of cardiovascular and non-cardiovascular multimorbidity after acute coronary syndrome. PLoS One. 2018;13(4):e0195174.

ACUTE CORONARY SYNDROME WITH COMORBIDITIES

The risk of death in patients of ACS with a comorbidity increases proportionately with incremental increase in CCI score. Similarly, the risk of death was almost two times more in patients with any comorbidity (CCI >0) when compared to patients with no comorbidity (CCI = 0).

Jeger et al. reported in an ACS registry that the incidence of major adverse cardiovascular events (MACEs) increased with a CCI score—equal to or more than 2 during a 1-year follow-up period after ACS.[4]

In yet another study, Nunez et al. revealed that a higher CCI score is an independent predictor of mortality or AMI at 30 days and 1 year.[5]

RELATIONSHIP OF COMORBIDITY AND STABLE HEART DISEASE

It was revealed in the meta-analysis by Rashid et al. that an incremental increase in CCI score is associated with increased mortality even in stable heart disease.[1]

PATIENTS UNDERGOING PERCUTANEOUS INTERVENTION

Majority of the studies looking into the long-term survival after PCI for CAD have reported increased mortality with each point increase in CCI score.[1]

The conclusion of the study by Rashid et al. reveals that association of comorbidity has an inverse relationship to the survival outcomes in patients with heart disease. This finding has important implications in management of heart disease. Since the noncardiovascular comorbidities are usually not factored into while calculating mortality and survival outcomes in CHD unlike the traditional comorbid conditions such as diabetes, hyperlipidemia, hypertension, the findings of the study by Rashid et al. carry important long-term implications.

The mechanism by which the comorbid conditions such as CKD, liver cirrhosis, cerebrovascular disease influence outcomes in CVD is complex and multifactorial. Moreover, older and frailer patients with a relatively higher burden of comorbidity are likely to be treated with increased caution and often unwarranted conservative approach unlike the younger patients with no comorbid condition. For instance, it was found in a large, national ACS registry that there was an incremental reduction in the provision of evidence-based treatments such as aspirin, statins, angiotensin-converting enzyme (ACE) inhibitors and reperfusion therapy in older patients with multiple comorbid conditions.[6] In another recent analysis involving 18,814 patients, Patel et al. reported that patients with comorbid burden, as defined by CCI score, were less likely to be offered coronary angiography and/or reperfusion therapy when presented with ST segment elevation myocardial infarction (STEMI).[7] In addition, in the setting of acute ischemic stroke, thrombolysis is often denied to older patients with comorbidities due to fear of hemorrhage unlike the younger patients with no comorbidity.[8] While managing chronic heart failure, deployment of ACE inhibitors and spironolactone is many a times withheld if there is a concurrent chronic kidney disease. Similarly, the treating physicians are often reluctant to use beta-blockers in elderly patients with chronic obstructive pulmonary disease.[9]

It is also true that aggressive treatment strategies in elderly patients with multiple comorbidities can result in adverse outcomes and heightened probability of complications. For instance, patients with leukemia are at an increased risk for in-stent thrombosis. Similarly, patients with liver cirrhosis have a greater likelihood of hemorrhage after PCI when antiplatelet agents are used. Consequently, the treating physicians face a daunting challenge to find a balance between the risks and benefits of a therapeutic intervention. The challenge is particularly stiff while managing patients with CHD and comorbidities in the present time because multiple treatment options such as medical therapies, PCI, surgical revascularization, device therapies and thrombolysis are now readily available to wider spectrum of patients.

The author has faced many such challenges in his daily practice. Through this book, author intend to help his colleagues in cardiology to live up to the difficult task of managing patients of heart disease harboring various comorbid conditions. The author had to sift through a large amount of available literature on this subject before presenting this book so that the reader can make management decisions that are evidence-based. The author intend to drive home the message that there must be a thorough assessment of the comorbid status in patients of heart disease and that the impact of comorbidity on long-term survival must be integrated into the counseling of such patients. Any choice of treatment must be preceded by assessment of comorbid conditions apart from traditional risk assessment.

REFERENCES

1. Rashid M, Kwok CS, Gale CP, et al. Impact of comorbid burden on mortality in patients with coronary heart disease, heart failure, and cerebrovascular accident: a systematic review and meta-analysis. Eur Heart J Qual Care Clin Outcomes. 2017;3:20-36.
2. Canivell S, Muller O, Gencer B, et al. Prognosis of cardiovascular and non-cardiovascular multimorbidity after acute coronary syndrome. PLoS One. 2018;13(4):e0195174.
3. Charlson ME, Pompei P, Ales KL, et al. A new method of classifying prognostic comorbidity in longitudinal studies: development and validation. J Chronic Dis. 1987;40: 373-83.
4. Jeger R, Jaguszewski M, Nallamothu BN, et al. Acute multivessel revascularization improves 1-year outcome in ST-elevation myocardial infarction: a nationwide study cohort from the AMIS Plus registry. Int J Cardiol. 2014;172:76-81.
5. Nunez JE, Nunez E, Facila L, et al. Prognostic value of Charlson comorbidity index at 30 days and 1 year after acute myocardial infarction. Rev Esp Cardiol. 2004;57:842-9.
6. Zaman MJ, Stirling S, Shepstone L, et al. The association between older age and receipt of care and outcomes in patients with acute coronary syndromes: a cohort study of the Myocardial Ischaemia National Audit Project (MINAP). Eur Heart J. 2014;35:1551-8.
7. Patel N, Patel NJ, Thakkar B, et al. Management strategies and outcomes of ST-segment elevation myocardial infarction patients transferred after receiving fibrinolytic therapy in the United States. Clin Cardiol. 2016;39:9-18.
8. Bateman BT, Schumacher HC, Boden-Albala B, et al. Factors associated with In-hospital mortality after administration of thrombolysis in acute ischemic stroke patients: an analysis of the nationwide inpatient sample 1999 to 2002. Stroke. 2006;37:440-6.
9. Muzzarelli S, Maeder MT, Toggweiler S, et al. Frequency and predictors of hyperkalemia in patients ≥60 years of age with heart failure undergoing intense medical therapy. Am J Cardiol. 2012;109:693-8.

CHAPTER 2

Acute Coronary Syndrome with Stroke

Prologue
Devil and the Deep Sea

On a cold December morning last year, a 62-year-old gentleman was admitted under my care complaining of a severe chest pain—suggesting acute coronary syndrome (ACS). He was a known to be suffering from high blood pressure (BP) and on medication. Since his baseline electrocardiogram (EKG or ECG) showed telltale signs of myocardial ischemia, the author decided to proceed with coronary angiography (CAG). A significant stenosis was detected in the left anterior descending artery (LAD) and left circumflex artery (LCX). The author reperfused the ischemic myocardium using drug-eluting stents (DESs) and started on dual antiplatelet therapy (DAPT). He was free of chest pain and his general condition showed a steady improvement. The author was planning to shift him from the intensive care unit (ICU) to the rooms the following day. However, on the 3rd day after angioplasty, this patient complained of a severe headache and his BP had shot up. The author deferred his plan to discharge the patient and asked for an emergency computed tomography (CT) scan of the brain instead. A moderate-sized and acute subarachnoid hemorrhage showed up on the CT scan. That explained the recent headache. The author was forced to stop the dual antiplatelet drugs. Neurologist did not feel any need of intervention and stated conservative treatment. Fortunately, he did not have significant neurodeficit and stabilized in couple of days. Five days later, he complained of severe chest pain again. On examination and ECG, he had suffered a massive ischemic infarction of the anterior wall of the left ventricle. A repeat coronary angiogram revealed exactly what the author feared the most—the cessation of DAPT had resulted in complete occlusion of the LAD due to stent thrombosis. Fortunately, the stent in the LCX was patent. Now, the author was staring at the proverbial situation of choosing between the devil and deep sea. If the author desisted from repeat angioplasty and thrombus aspiration for the fear of increasing the size of a 3-day old intracranial hematoma, this patient would probably die due to the massive myocardial infarction (MI) and its complications. On the contrary, if the author proceeded with the angioplasty, which required anticoagulation and antiplatelets, and there was a theoretical possibility of an increase in the size of the intracerebral hemorrhage (ICH) or even a fresh hemorrhage at a different site—jeopardizing his life. The author chose the former option and went ahead with thrombus aspiration, balloon angioplasty and gave a single shot of 5,000 units of heparin and started only aspirin. And, the author prayed! As luck would have it, this gentleman survived with no further complications. His chest pain was relieved and the next couple of days in the ICU were uneventful—allowing me to discharge him from the hospital a few days later.

Last month, another 70-year-old man came under my care with complaints of chest pain. His baseline cardiac workup confirmed the diagnosis of infarction of the anterior myocardial wall of the left ventricle. Since he had complained of a transient giddiness and slurring of speech earlier, the author asked for a CT scan followed by magnetic resonance imaging (MRI) of the brain. The imaging studies revealed a small-sized and acute lacunar infarct. Since the infarct size was small, intravascular thrombolysis was not contemplated. The treating neurologist was not in favor of a percutaneous coronary intervention (PCI) for the acute myocardial infarction (MI) because he feared the cerebral infarct may end up with a hemorrhagic conversion due to the antiplatelet therapy given after the angioplasty. The author and his colleague decided to wait and treat the MI with medication alone for the time being. A week later, the author went ahead with the coronary angiogram, which revealed a significant stenosis of the LAD. The author proceeded with the angioplasty using a DES, anticoagulation with 5,000 units of heparin, and DAPT (ticagrelor and aspirin). This patient did well and his further stay in the hospital was uneventful. He is still on DAPT and he continues to be well on follow-up period.

■ INTRODUCTION

Acute ischemic stroke (AIS) and acute myocardial infarction (AMI) are potentially life-threatening medical conditions. If not recognized and treated promptly, both these conditions carry a grave prognosis. When an infarction of one vascular territory precedes infarction in another vascular territory, the presentation is called as "metachronous presentation". In the past, several scientific studies have highlighted an association between AIS and AMI. For instance, a 3-year prospective study of patients admitted with symptoms of AIS in a geriatric unit[1] showed that 12.7% of them developed an associated AMI within 72 hours after hospitalization.

Even though AIS and AMI result from sudden and complete occlusion of the feeding arteries, important differences exist in their pathophysiology, subsequent course, and management. Firstly, AIS results from distal emboli,[2] while AMI is caused by local thrombus.[3] Material composition of the distal emboli causing AIS is different from the local thrombi leading to AMI.[4,5] The chemical composition along with fibrinolytic and mechanical properties of the distal emboli affects the site and distribution of ischemia in the brain tissue.[6] Secondly, in view of development of vasogenic edema and probable intraparenchymal hemorrhage, damage to the blood–brain barrier that happens in AIS is far more detrimental[7,8] when compared to the relatively less deleterious endothelial damage occurring due to the local thrombi in coronary arteries.[9] Thirdly, the network of collateral vessels in the brain is much more efficient than the similar network in myocardium.[10-13] Fourthly, the topography and size of the ischemic lesion in the brain determine the prognosis,[14] while in ST elevation myocardial infarction (STEMI), size of the ischemic lesion alone determines the final outcome.

Over the years, awareness about metachronous presentation of AIS and AMI has increased leading to much more coherent and efficient management of the two conditions. AIS and AMI have a narrow time window for therapy so much, so that acute management of one condition at the expense of the other condition usually results in an irreversible damage. In addition, the standard use of antiplatelets and anticoagulant drugs during and after percutaneous intervention in MI may increase the probability of hemorrhagic conversion of an ischemic infarct in the brain, especially when it is treated with intravascular thrombolysis.[15,16] Similarly, use of thrombolytic agents in AIS increases the possibility of a rupture of the infarcted cardiac wall in AMI. As per the guidelines for early management of AIS, use of thrombolytic agents is a contraindication if the patient has suffered AMI during the 3 months prior to the event.[17] Similarly, thrombolysis is contraindicated in AMI with prior hemorrhagic stroke or ischemic stroke in prior 1 year.

■ DEFINITION OF CARDIOCEREBRAL INFARCTION—NEW TERMINOLOGY

In the year 2010, Omar et al. presented a case report of "cardiocerebral infarction", which is simultaneous AIS and MI.[18] Reported incidence of simultaneous cardiocerebral infarction is 0.009%.[19]

The term "synchronous cardiocerebral infarction" is used to describe the simultaneous ischemic event in cerebral and cardiac vascular territories while the term "metachronous cardiocerebral infarction" is used to describe the cases when infarction in one territory precedes infarction in other territory.

Many studies have shown that AIS increases the risk for AMI and vice-versa.[20,21] However, simultaneous occurrence of AIS and AMI, which used to be called earlier as "cardiocerebral infarction", is reported rarely.[18] Proposed new term for this condition is "hyperacute simultaneous cardiocerebral infarction". This term is used to describe the patients with simultaneous cardiocerebral infarction who arrived at the hospital within the recommended therapeutic window of 4.5 hours after the onset of symptoms. Management of this rare condition is a challenging task, especially because there are no ideal and recommended guidelines for treatment. Primary aim of management of this condition is to salvage, as much as possible, the noninfarcted and viable brain or heart tissue.

EPIDEMIOLOGY OF ISCHEMIC STROKE AND MYOCARDIAL INFARCTION

Many observational and prospective studies, done as early as 1970, have reported an association between the cerebrovascular disease and coronary artery disease (CAD). A prospective study by Rokey et al.[8] reported the prevalence of CAD as 58% among the patients presenting with transient ischemic attacks (TIAs) as well as AIS. As per the Austrian Stroke Unit Registry, 1% of the patients with TIA or AIS and 0.3% of the patients with cerebral hemorrhage developed MI during their stay in the hospital.[22] Similarly, several studies have reported occurrence as well as increased risk of a cerebrovascular accident after a cardiac event.[21,23,24] These studies have reported 0.9% incidence of in-hospital stroke in patients hospitalized for acute coronary syndrome (ACS), especially STEMI.

PATHOPHYSIOLOGY OF SIMULTANEOUS CARDIOCEREBRAL INFARCTION

Pathophysiology of cardiocerebral infarction can be classified into following three categories:
1. Conditions leading to concurrent cerebral and MI
2. Cardiac conditions leading to cerebral infarction
3. Brain–heart axis dysregulation (cerebral infarction) leading to MI.

Atrial fibrillation is reported to lead to concurrent cerebral and MI. In this condition, the intracardiac emboli are thought to be the common source of occlusion of cerebral and coronary vessels.[25,26] In Type I aortic dissection, the intimal flap can extend into the coronary as well as cerebral arteries leading to concurrent cerebral and MI.[27] Electrocution injury leading to diffuse spasm of the cerebral and coronary arteries is thought to be a rare cause of simultaneous cardiocerebral infarction.[28] In left ventricular dysfunction with poor ejection fraction, pre-existing intracardiac thrombi can result in cardiocerebral infarction. Similarly, a right ventricular failure and thrombus formation associated with patent foramen ovale may lead to simultaneous occlusion of the cerebral and coronary arteries.[18] Severe hypotension after an AMI can result in marked hypoperfusion of the brain and subsequently infarction of the brain tissue.[18,19]

The brain–heart axis dysregulation that happens in cerebral infarction may be another alternative source of simultaneous cardiocerebral infarction. The parietoinsular cortex of the brain is thought to regulate the autonomic nervous system. An ischemic injury to this area may result in sympathetic overactivity and subsequent myocardial injury (myocytolysis) confirmed by elevated serum levels of cardiac enzymes, cardiac arrhythmias, and disruption of diurnal variation of BP.[29] Stimulation of the insular cortex in right cerebral hemisphere is known to have predominant sympathetic effect, while the same cortex in left hemisphere is known to have a predominant parasympathetic effect.[29,30] In one study, abnormalities on ECG including ST segment elevation and increased serum levels of cardiac troponin T were shown to be associated with an ischemic infarction of the parietoinsular cortex of the brain.[30]

■ HYPERACUTE SIMULTANEOUS CARDIOCEREBRAL INFARCTION: MANAGEMENT AND DILEMMA

A case of hyperacute simultaneous cardiocerebral infarction presents enormous challenge and dilemma to the treating physician. Dependable recommendations for optimal reperfusion strategy in the setting of cardiocerebral infarction are lacking because of its rarity. The main dilemma is that initial treatment of one condition results in inevitable delay in addressing the other problem. Intravenous (IV) thrombolytic therapy with recombinant tissue plasminogen activator (rtPA) is a standard and universally prescribed treatment regimen for the patients with AIS who present to the hospital within 4.5 hours after the onset of symptoms (Table 1).[17] Primary percutaneous coronary intervention (PCI) is the first-line therapy for the patients presenting with STEMI as well as non-ST elevation acute coronary syndromes (NSTE-ACS).[31,32] Fibrinolytic therapy within 12 hours after the onset of angina is an alternative treatment method, especially where facility for primary PCI is unavailable. However, this is not recommended in the setting of NSTE-ACS because of the increased risk of intracranial hemorrhage and MI.[32] A scientific statement coming from American Heart Association/American Stroke Association (AHA/ASA) states that in a setting of hyperacute cardiocerebral infarction, IV alteplase in suitable dose for cerebral ischemia followed by percutaneous angioplasty and stenting is reasonable.[33] Therapy with fibrinolytic agents such as IV rtPA can be used to treat AIS and also acute STEMI. However, significant differences in dose requirements and timing of fibrinolytic therapy hinder the use of IV rtPA as a definitive treatment for these conditions.[33] Moreover, higher dose and longer infusion time of rtPA required to treat STEMI in comparison with the dose required to treat AIS may increase the likelihood of hemorrhagic transformation of a concurrent cerebral ischemic infarct.[31,33] The AHA/ASA recommendation is silent on management of subtypes of AMI. Even though an AMI has a longer therapeutic window for reperfusion when compared to cerebral infarction, an urgent institution of appropriate reperfusion therapy is desirable. A delay in reperfusion of ischemic myocardium may lead to hemodynamic instability and other cardiac complications including hemopericardium, cardiac rupture, and tamponade.

The ultimate aim of treatment in metachronous as well as synchronous cardiocerebral infarction is to reperfuse the cardiac and cerebral tissue at risk in a timely fashion, so that irreversible damage to either tissue is prevented. A meta-analysis, which looked at five randomized trials (of ischemic stroke) comparing IV thrombolysis alone versus in combination with endovascular therapy following IV thrombolysis, concluded that combination therapy was better in improving functional independency with number needed to treat (NNT) of 2.6. Thus, a combined treatment of IV thrombolysis followed by endovascular treatment is recommended for ischemic stroke due to large vessel occlusion.[34]

Following is the course of treatment in cardiocerebral infarction when a patient presents within 4.5 hours after the onset of stroke and develops a metachronous MI within 12 hours after the hospitalization.

An accurate evaluation of the hemodynamic stability at the time of initial presentation will help to decide the line of management. Once the clinical assessment of hemodynamic stability is done, a CT brain followed by CT angiography and CT perfusion study is recommended along with an ECG. If the patient is hemodynamically unstable and/or STEMI is diagnosed on ECG, an emergency PCI is the first choice of treatment. If the patient is stable hemodynamically and if there is no STEMI, IV infusion of fibrinolytic agents (rtPA) in the standard dose of 0.9 mg/kg body weight is suggested. Alternatively tenectaplase can be used though it is yet to be approved by FDA (Table 1). If the CT angiography followed by CT perfusion shows occlusion of a large vessel [carotid artery or stem of middle cerebral artery (MCA)] and if there is a perfusion mismatch, endovascular treatment for stroke is recommended along with primary PCI for STEMI. If the large cerebral vessels are patent and if there is no perfusion mismatch on CT perfusion study, medical management of the stroke will suffice. Many studies[35,36] have shown that infarction of insular cortex in right cerebral hemisphere due to occlusion of MCA has a higher mortality because of the sympathetic overactivity leading to cardiac arrhythmia. Hence, detection of a right MCA territory infarction on CT brain with angiogram warrants a close monitoring for cardiac arrhythmias. In the absence of right MCA infarction, a selective PCI is recommended to reperfuse the concurrent ischemic myocardium. This is combined with medical management of the stroke and AMI with dual antiplatelet therapy.

■ PRIOR STROKE AND ACUTE CORONARY SYNDROME

Approximately 5–10% of the patients presenting with AMI have a prior history of ischemic or hemorrhagic stroke.[2] This study also reveals that prior stroke is common in patients with non-STEMI (NSTEMI) rather than STEMI.[2] This finding is on the expected lines because patients with NSTEMI are more likely to be older and have atherosclerotic disease in the vessels. The demographic differences and likely history of diabetes explain the differences in use and outcome of PCI and medication between patients with prior history of stroke and those without such a history.[37-39] Considering the increased risk of poor outcome in patients with prior history of stroke, it is reasonable to expect that this group of patients are

TABLE 1: Comparing commonly used fibrinolytic agents.

Agent	US FDA-approved indication	Dose	Comments
Alteplase	Acute ischemic stroke (AIS)	0.1 mg/kg bolus followed by 0.8 mg/kg infusion over 60 min	ICH 0.4–0.6% maximum 90 mg in stroke
	STEMI	Total dose 100 mg [(15 mg bolus over 1–2 min) 0.75 mg/kg over 30 min (maximum 50 mg) 0.5 mg/kg over 60 min (maximum 35 mg) 2 min]	Fibrin specific
	Pulmonary embolism (PE)	100 mg over 2 h	Fibrinogen sparing
Reteplase	STEMI	10 mg push over 2 min repeat after 30 min	Anaphylaxis ICH 0.8%
Tenecteplase	STEMI	30–50 mg IV bolus for weight <60 kg to >90 kg	Most fibrin specific, fibrinogen sparing
	AIS (not FDA approved)	0.25 mg/kg maximum 25 mg bolus	ICH 0.9%
			More effective than alteplase in one trial
Streptokinase	STEMI	1.5 million units over 60 min	Anaphylaxis
	Acute PE/DVT	250,000 units over 30 min then	ICH not reported
		100,000 units/hour over 24 h (PE) or 72 h (DVT)	

(DVT: deep vein thrombosis; ICH: intracerebral hemorrhage; STEMI: ST elevation myocardial infarction; FDA: Food and Drug Administration)

more likely to benefit from evidence-based interventional procedures and medication. However, on the contrary, many studies have revealed that patients with previous history of stroke are less likely to receive reperfusion therapies and medications like aspirin and statins with proven efficacy. Global Registry of Acute Coronary Events (GRACE) clearly documents that reperfusion therapies are underutilized in older patients; women and patients with previous history of diabetes or heart failure in spite of the prevailing evidence that these patients would benefit from such therapies.[40] Even after adjusting for the demographic factors of age and gender, patients with prior history of stroke are still less likely to receive primary PCI when presented with AMI or ACS.

A review of 3,893 patients who underwent PCI between June, 2003 and September, 2005 in a hospital in Beijing, China discovered no significant difference in major adverse cardiac and cerebrovascular events (MACCEs) between the patients with prior history of stroke and those with no such prior history.[41] In this study, patients with prior stroke had frequent high-risk baseline features like diabetes, hypertension, hyperlipidemia and prior MI. The patients with prior history of stroke in this study had the stroke at least 3 months prior to the presentation to hospital with MI.

STROKE AFTER PERCUTANEOUS CORONARY INTERVENTION

Stroke after PCI is not common as revealed by an analysis of half a million patients undergoing PCI in a national PCI database in the United Kingdom, by Myint et al.[42] However, 30-day mortality and major adverse cardiovascular event (MACE) are high once the stroke occurs. Surprisingly, Phyo et al. discovered that odds of complications are higher in patients subjected to elective PCI when compared to the patients with ACS undergoing primary PCI. According to this study, the reason for this rather surprising finding is that patients with ACS undergoing primary PCI were treated with newer and more potent antiplatelet agents such as ticagrelor, prasugrel and glycoprotein IIb/IIIa inhibitors. On the contrary, in view of the lower risk profile, the patients subjected to elective PCI were treated with clopidogrel at the time of procedure. The potent antiplatelet drugs given to the patients in ACS groups had a protective effect against ischemic cerebral infarcts but the down side being increased incidence of fatal hemorrhagic stroke.

STROKE IN CATHETERIZATION LABORATORY DURING PERCUTANEOUS CORONARY INTERVENTION

Incidence

It is known that risk factors for cerebral stroke and CAD are similar. Therefore, it is expected that patients undergoing intervention for CAD are likely to suffer a periprocedural stroke. However, it is not a common experience. Incidence of stroke during or immediately after a diagnostic cardiac catheterization procedure ranges from 0.11% to 0.4%, while the same figures during or after PCI range from 0.18% to 0.44%. Incidence of a hemorrhagic stroke after a PCI procedure is marginally higher and slated to be 0.2–0.3%.[43-49] These figures highlight the fact that, though rare, stroke does occur either during or after a percutaneous intervention for a CAD. The duration of hospital stay for these patients increases and so is the likelihood of a persistent disability after the discharge. The in-hospital mortality rate in patients suffering from this complication ranges from 25% to 44%.[48,49] Hence, it is imperative that the staff working in a cardiac catheterization laboratory (CCL) is sensitized to detect and treat this potentially catastrophic complication in a time-bound manner. Establishing clear protocols in place will help early detection and prompt management.

Symptoms

Symptoms of stroke vary and depend on extent and location of the infarct or hemorrhage. In general population, strokes are common in the territory of anterior circulation (middle and anterior cerebral artery). However, strokes occurring as a complication of PCI tend to affect the vertebrobasilar circulation more often. Since 20% of the total cerebral blood flow runs through the posterior circulation, even a small infarct or hemorrhage in this area can result in a significant and potentially fatal neurodeficit.[49,50] Facial paresthesia, sudden sensorineural hearing loss, dysarthria, dysphagia and hemisensory defects in the extremities are some of the common symptoms experienced by the patients who have a posterior circulation stroke. The other common symptoms are motor or speech deficits, aphasia, change in mental status and visual disturbances. Some of the symptoms can be camouflaged, if the patient is sedated. It is important to remember that seizures, hypoglycemia, and migraine can mimic symptoms of stroke. Moreover, the so-called "silent" infarcts or asymptomatic infarcts are not reflected in the statistics quoted for periprocedural stroke. The patients with "silent" infarcts may have no symptoms at all or they may have minor cognitive deficits. Reported incidence of asymptomatic cerebral infarcts during or after a PCI is approximately 15%.[48,51]

Pathophysiology

The chemical composition of the emboli causing stroke is variable. These emboli can consist of air, soft clot, calcified atheroma, or an atheroma with a fibrin clot around it. Since the catheters used for PCI have a larger caliber and stiffer than those used for diagnostic catheterization, possibility of dislodging an atheroma along the aortic walls during manipulation is higher. The thrombus formed at the catheter tip can also be the source of emboli.[45,48,52,53] The likelihood of emboli leading to stroke is more, if a transradial approach is employed instead of the usual transfemoral approach for catheterization.[45,48]

Management

Brain tissue has minimal oxygen reserves and cannot withstand an ischemic situation for long. Therefore, it is imperative that reperfusion therapy is initiated without any undue delay in order to prevent permanent disability and death. Appropriate treatment must be initiated within 60 minutes after the patient's arrival in the emergency department or the discovery of symptoms of stroke in the CCL. An emergency CT scan must be ordered to differentiate an ischemic stroke from cerebral hemorrhage. Once the ischemic stroke is confirmed, the treating neurologist must weigh the benefits versus risks of different treatment strategies and formulate a plan for management. If the patient's condition and type of infarct meet the criteria for IV fibrinolysis therapy, tissue plasminogen activator (tPA) must be started immediately.

If necessary, an interventional neurologist or a radiologist can perform relevant intravascular intervention after a digital subtraction angiogram (DSA). The dosage of IV tPA is weight-dependent and the prescribed dosage is 0.9 mg/kg to a maximum of 90 mg. The drug is mixed in sterile water and must not be shaken or sent through a pneumatic. IV tPA is administered in two stages—10% of the total dose is given through a dedicated IV line over 1 minute followed by administration of remaining 90% of the dose over 60 minutes through an infusion pump.

During IV infusion of tPA, patient must be closely monitored in an intensive care unit (ICU) for any signs of complications—mainly cerebral hemorrhage. Vital signs should be assessed and neurological examination must be done every 15 minutes for 2 hours, every half hour for 6 hours, and finally every hour for next 16 hours. In 5% of the patients receiving IV tPA, complications occur.[48] Intracranial or systemic hemorrhage and angioedema are two of the feared complications of tPA administration. These require immediate intervention. Retroperitoneal hemorrhage and groin hematoma can also occur. It is advisable to leave the sheath in place for several hours when stroke occurs during PCI. It helps to minimize the risk of hemorrhage due to IV tPA. In case of a hemorrhagic stroke, anticoagulation must be discontinued and a neurosurgeon should be consulted to determine whether surgical intervention is necessary. Hyperbaric oxygen therapy and 100% oxygen by face mask is advised, if the stroke is due to air embolism.

■ PERCUTANEOUS CORONARY INTERVENTION IN ACUTE STROKE

Cardiac events like ACS and AMI are frequent in patients with acute stroke. An emergency PCI in AMI has a proven value in improving the outcome. However, the treatment scenario in a synchronous or metachronous cardiocerebral infarction is more complex because medication with blood-thinning, clot-busting drugs are indispensable during and after PCI and these very drugs are contraindicated when there is a concomitant hemorrhagic stroke. In addition, when administered in an inappropriate dose for a variable duration, these drugs can result in hemorrhagic transformation of an ischemic stroke. A single-center and case-series study was conducted with the aim to investigate safety of PCI in 80 patients hospitalized with AIS and a concomitant ACS.[54] Patients with TIAs were also included in the study. Patients who underwent subsequent PCI were compared with those who were treated with medications alone. The primary endpoint in this study was a mixture of death, recurrent MI, coronary reintervention, recurrent stroke, and systemic hemorrhage during 1-year follow-up period. The primary endpoint during the 1-year follow-up period did not differ in the two groups. Incidence of intracerebral bleed was lower in the group who underwent PCI.

STROKE AFTER PRIMARY ANGIOPLASTY IN MYOCARDIAL INFARCTION

An analytical study was done by Guptill et al. to assess the incidence, type and timing of stroke, and prespecified 90-day clinical outcomes in stroke after Primary Angioplasty in Myocardial Infarction (PAMI).[55] They studied 5,372 patients enrolled in the Assessment of Pexelizumab in Acute Myocardial Infarction (APEX-AMI) trial. They found that stroke occurred in 69 patients (1.3%) who underwent primary PCI. A third of these strokes were ischemic, 12% were hemorrhagic strokes, while the remaining 55% were of indeterminate type. The medial time of stroke occurrence was 6, 101 and 102 days, respectively. Overall, 43% of the strokes occurred within 48 hours after PCI and all the hemorrhagic strokes occurred within 48 hours. Stroke was associated with an increased risk of 90-day death, congestive heart failure (CHF), and 30-day hospital readmission. Since most of the strokes occurred 48 hours after PCI, this study concluded that not all the strokes after primary PCI are procedure related and that some other mechanisms may be responsible for the later events. A relatively high proportion of the hemorrhagic strokes in patients who received glycoprotein IIb/IIIa inhibitors suggest that special attention must be paid to this particular class of drugs in patients undergoing primary PCI for STEMI. However, whether hemorrhagic strokes can be prevented by carefully avoiding over anticoagulation still needs to be proven.

A recent meta-analysis of trials evaluating the use of thrombus aspiration devices has found that these devices caused 2.8-fold increase in the incidence of stroke even while increasing myocardial tissue perfusion.[56] This study suggests careful engagement and repeated aspiration of the guide catheter to minimize the risk of adverse events during aspiration of thrombus by aspiration devices and primary PCI. Large myocardial infarcts in patients with STEMI are known to result in clot formation within left ventricles during first 24 hours. Such clot formation can be significantly reduced with anticoagulation.

STROKE DURING THE PERIOD AFTER MYOCARDIAL INFARCTION

Newer pharmacological agents and mechanical interventions have significantly improved chances of survival after a MI. However, stroke continues to be a potentially catastrophic complication after STEMI as well as NSTE-ACS. Mortality due to stroke after an MI is up to 60% at 1 year.[57,58] Mortality rate from an ischemic stroke is up to 10–20% while mortality from a hemorrhagic stroke is higher. When compared with a matched cohort of stroke patients with no preceding MI, patients with stroke after a MI had a higher rate of in-hospital and long-term mortality of 30% and residual deficits at 6 months.[59]

Incidence of Stroke during the Post-MI Period

A recent community-based study of stroke incidence after MI[60] found a 44-fold increase in risk of stroke within first 3 months after MI and the risk persisted even 3 years later. As per this study, advancements in therapy have not changed mortality during post-MI period. The participants of this study were followed for a period of a decade and even longer.

Nearly 10 million (1,000,000) individuals are diagnosed with AMI during 1 year in the United States of America. In view of such a large number of patients with MI, risk of stroke after MI is substantial.[61] The incidence of an ischemic stroke within a month after a STEMI is found to be 2%, while the same risk after NSTE-ACS is 1%.[62-64] However, the level of risk of an individual patient can be determined better based on presence or absence of certain clinical factors like age >75 years, black race, diabetes, hypertension, atrial fibrillation, peripheral vascular disease, etc.[65] In the patients of STEMI treated with fibrinolytics, most ischemic strokes occur 48 hours after the cardiac event. In any case, the first 28 days after a STEMI is the most vulnerable period for an ischemic stroke.[66]

Pathogenesis of Stroke after Myocardial Infarction

Historic view has been that myocardial injury suffered during a large infarct alters flow characteristics leading to the formation of left ventricular mural thrombus (LVMT), which in turn become a potential source of embolic events. Therefore, systemic anticoagulation is thought to be protective.[67] The LVMT is thought to occur by 2 weeks after an MI in 0.6–3.7% of the patients. However, this rate is substantially lower than the reported earlier incidence of 20–56%.[68] Adjunctive therapies with antiplatelet agents and antithrombotic agents combined with early revascularization might have contributed to this reduction of formation of LVMT and subsequent embolic events. An alternative mechanism is described for the pathogenesis of stroke after MI. Tendency for increased coagulation during an ACS is known to persist for at least 6 months and it has the potential for thromboembolic events and stroke.[69] Emboli can come from aorta, carotid arteries, left atrium, or left ventricle. Activation of catecholamine during an ACS may lead to enhanced platelet aggregation and thrombus formation. A heightened state of inflammation persists in the coronary arteries after an ACS. The circulating inflammatory cytokines may trigger a cascade of events in the cerebral circulation as well. Complex and unstable plaques are common in the carotid arteries after an ACS.[70] These unstable plaques can rupture and result in thromboembolic events in cerebral circulation.

The technology of mechanical revascularization of occluded coronary arteries has seen a rapid advancement in recent years. Similarly, efficacy of adjunctive pharmacological agents has improved. As a result, PCI has become a standard of acre and more and more people are undergoing cardiac catheterization and revascularization whenever indicated. It has improved outcomes in high-risk patients with ACS. However, the net effect of these developments in the overall incidence of stroke is worrisome. GUSTO-1[71] data showed that coronary angiography (CAG) and coronary artery bypass graft surgery (CABG) were associated with increased risk of stroke. An analysis of OASIS (Organization to Assess Strategies for Ischemic Syndromes) registry showed patients from countries with higher rates of CABG and CAG suffered an increased risk of stroke at 6 months.[72] However, in a more recent analysis, OASIS patient, only CABG, was associated with heightened risk of stroke and no significant risk of stroke was found in patients undergoing PCI.[58] The type of revascularization therapy can influence the risk of stroke in the setting of ACS.[73] The 6-month incidence of stroke among NSTE-ACS patients undergoing PCI was lower when compared to patients treated with CABG.[58]

ANTIPLATELET THERAPY

Treatment with aspirin therapy is the single most effective antiplatelet therapy in prevention of ischemic stroke after an MI. It is now a universal practice to prescribe at least 81 mg of aspirin daily to all patients with MI unless there is a definite allergy. However, with the increasing use of PCI to treat patients with AMI, combination of clopidogrel, which is an adenosine diphosphate (ADP) receptor antagonist, with aspirin has become widespread. However, CURE trial[74] of long-term clopidogrel in addition to aspirin showed insignificant reduction in incidence of stroke. The minimal benefit was hampered by increased risk of ICH due to combination therapy. Similarly, the MATCH trial[75] showed increased risk of intracerebral bleed when clopidogrel was used in combination with aspirin rather than when it was given alone.

ANTICOAGULATION THERAPY

Anticoagulation agents, such as heparins, form the cornerstone of pharmacological treatment of patients with ACS. Rebound increase in thrombotic events is reported after cessation of heparin therapy.[76] Several post-MI trials[77-81] have compared aspirin alone versus aspirin–warfarin combination to prevent ischemic stroke after an MI (STEMI as well as NSTE-ACS). Most of these trials have favored warfarin with aspirin or warfarin alone. However, low-dose warfarin (INR 2–3) as well as high-dose warfarin (INR 1–2.8) has an increased tendency to cause cerebral hemorrhage. Thus, warfarin at a moderate dose with INR 2–3 along with aspirin (75–162 mg) appears to be more effective in reducing strokes after ACS when compared to aspirin alone. However, this regimen comes at a cost of some increase in the likelihood of bleeding. All subsets of ACS patients appear to benefit from this combination therapy.

Since all current revascularization therapies for MI support the use of combination of aspirin and clopidogrel during the weeks and months after

MI, primary question involves the risk and benefit of additional protection against thrombotic events. Role of warfarin in clinical scenarios like atrial fibrillation and left ventricular mural thrombosis is well established and warfarin is clearly superior to combination of aspirin with clopidogrel. However, triple therapy, consisting of aspirin, clopidogrel, and warfarin, in the setting of coronary stenting puts these patients at increased risk of bleeding. Patients with increased risk of bleeding must receive triple therapy with close monitoring of INR and for the least possible duration (1–2 weeks for bare metal stents) followed by aspirin and warfarin combination. Irrespective of the method of anticoagulation, early treatment and timely revascularization are the best way to avoid a peri-MI stroke. If surgical revascularization is required in a stable patient, it is prudent to wait for at least 14 days for the CABG to minimize risk of a thromboembolic stroke.[58]

Safety of Abciximab Administration during Percutaneous Coronary Intervention of Patients with Previous Stroke

A database review of 7,244 consecutive PCI procedures from 7/97 to 10/01 was done.[82] This review identified 6,190 PCIs performed with abciximab among whom 515 patients had a prior stroke. Out of them, 101 patients had a recent ischemic stroke or an intracerebral bleed while 414 patients had a remote (>2 years prior) ischemic stroke. As per this database review, incidence of post-PCI stroke was significantly higher in patients who suffered a stroke earlier. This review revealed that incidence of intracerebral hematoma did not increase in patients who were treated with abciximab.

Ticagrelor versus Clopidogrel in PCI with Prior Stroke

Presently, it is not certain whether ticagrelor offers any mortality benefit.[83] However, when compared to patients with prior stroke and treated with clopidogrel, patients on ticagrelor are at a 2-fold increased risk of recurrent stroke or TIA and a 2-fold increased risk of intracranial hemorrhage.[84] Thus in patients with a history of CVD, ticagrelor does not have any net clinical benefit over clopidogrel. On the contrary, ticagrelor seems to carry a net clinical harm.

■ HEPARIN IN STROKE

Available data suggest that:
- In most patients with embolic cerebral infarcts, heparin-related hemorrhage occurs early less than 72 hours of stroke onset and within 24 hours after heparinization
- Intracerebral hemorrhage may follow heparinization in patients with moderate-sized or large cerebral infarcts and who have been anti-

coagulated earlier with activated partial thromboplastin time (APTT) more than twice the control
- Pathogenesis of intracranial hemorrhage is related to the phenomenon of hemorrhagic transformation of an ischemic infarct.

ANTICOAGULATION AND ANTIPLATELET TREATMENT IN INTRACRANIAL HEMORRHAGE

Hematoma Expansion

Expansion of intracerebral hemorrhage after presentation is fairly common. This is particularly observed in patients on antithrombotic therapy and is associated with worse prognosis. This may occur in first 24 hours in 15–38% of patients as observed by serial CT scans. The hematoma growth may be as high as more than 33% volume increase.[85] Subsequent incidence of hematoma between 24 hours is just 1–2%.[85] Persistent increased BP,, use of antithrombotic therapy, large size of hematoma, and spot sign (evidence of contrast extravasation on initial CT imaging) are some of the risk factors for hematoma expansion.

All antiplatelet and anticoagulant drugs should be immediately discontinued after the onset of ICH, and anticoagulant effect should be reversed immediately with appropriate reversing agents.

Anticoagulation (if absolutely indicated)

Paciaroni et al. in their meta-analysis of controlled studies looked at safety and efficacy of anticoagulation for prevention of venous thromboembolism in acute hemorrhagic stroke patients. They observed that, while early anticoagulation significantly reduces incidence of pulmonary thromboembolism, increase in hematoma size was not significant.[86]

As per the recommendation of American Heart Association/American Stroke Association Stroke Council guideline, as soon as intracranial bleeding cessation is documented, heparin, either low-molecular weight heparin (LMWH) or unfractionated, may be considered for deep vein thrombosis (DVT) or pulmonary embolism (PE) prophylaxis in those at high risk for it and may be started even as early as after 1st day of ICH onset.

As such as chances of hematoma expansion diminish after first couple of days, heparin may be used after 4 days of ICH, if its benefit outweighs the risk of hemorrhage worsening as in case of emergency PCI for ACS.

Antiplatelet Treatment in Intracerebral Hemorrhage

Aspirin and other antiplatelet therapies have been proven to be of benefit for secondary and, in some cases, primary prevention of ischemic events like ischemic stroke or MI. Over the years, prevalence of ischemic cardiac or brain diseases is increasing, especially in the elderly population. These diseases have high-recurrence rate necessitating continued usage of antiplatelet treatment for secondary prevention.

Antiplatelet treatment affects the platelet functioning thereby can predispose to spontaneous bleeding or affect the hemostatic function after occurrence of the bleeding event.

This was corroborated by a systemic review by McQuaid et al. They observed that treatment with antiplatelet agent increases the risk of hemorrhage including intracranial bleed.[87] Thus, antiplatelet treatment is relatively contraindicated in patients with primary intracranial hemorrhage, as they can increase the bleed size or promote recurrence and hence increasing morbidity or mortality. This has led the treating clinicians to adopt a very cautious approach in starting or resuming antiplatelet treatment in the patients who have ICH and who also need antiplatelet treatment. This will have serious implications in patients with ischemic heart disease or ischemic stroke wherein antiplatelet treatment is the cornerstone. Some studies have tried to address this therapeutic dilemma. Ding et al. in their extensive search of major databases found only six relevant cohort studies with 1,916 patients in total.[88] These studies have tried to assess the risk of restarting antiplatelet treatment in the patients with ICH. In their meta-analysis of these studies, Ding et al. observed a significant reduction of risk of ischemic and thromboembolic events after resumption of antiplatelet treatment. More importantly, there was no significant increase in either hematoma expansion or subsequent ICH recurrence in patients in whom antiplatelet treatment was resumed. Although this evidence should increase the confidence of treating clinician to start antiplatelets in those who absolutely need it, yet in any individual patient, risk-benefit ratio needs to be ascertained before taking a decision. Addressing the modifiable risk factor like control of BP and proper assessment of other bleeding risks may help to identify those patients in whom treatment benefit will outweigh the risk.

Timing of Resumption of Antiplatelet Therapy

Patient population, in whom antiplatelet treatment resumption is crucial, is those who have undergone recent PCI. The data is scarce in providing evidence of the proper time after ICH to resume antiplatelet treatment. Obviously one has to strike a balance between the risk of hematoma expansion in those who receive antiplatelets versus stent thrombosis in those who do not. Some quantifiable risk metric like ICH score might be useful in this regard. ICH score (0–6) utilizes the following parameters—the Glasgow Coma Scale on admission, ICH volume, infratentorial origin of the ICH, intraventricular hemorrhage on CT scan, and age. This score can assist in prediction of mortality in patients with ICH.[89] Hemphill et al. have underscored the value of this score by reporting a 30-day mortality of 0%, 13%, 26%, 72%, 97% and 100% when the ICH score was 0, 1, 2, 3, 4 and 5, respectively.[89] Similarly, the risk of stent thrombosis may be assessed by using various scores like DAPT score (Box 1).[90]

> **BOX 1** Variables used to calculate DAPT Score, are as follows with designated points.[90]
>
> - Age ≥75 years: -2
> - Age 65 to <75 years: -1
> - Age <65 years: 0
> - Current cigarette smoker: 1
> - Diabetes mellitus: 1
> - MI at presentation: 1
> - Prior PCI or prior MI: 1
> - Stent diameter <3 mm: 1
> - Paclitaxel-eluting stent: 1
> - CHF or LVEF <30%: 2
> - Saphenous vein graft PCI: 2
>
> *Note:* A score of ≥2 is associated with a favorable benefit–risk ratio for prolonged DAPT, while a score of <2 is associated with an unfavorable benefit–risk ratio.
>
> (CHF: congestive heart failure; DAPT: dual antiplatelet therapy; LVEF: left ventricular ejection fraction; MI: myocardial infarction; PCI: percutaneous coronary intervention)

Comparing the two scores, risk-benefit of resumption and timing of resumption of antiplatelet treatment may be decided. Though this strategy is general, when an individual patient is managed; beside this risk-benefit assessment, input from a multidisciplinary team of all treating physicians, patient and the family is required before taking a final call for starting antiplatelets and its timing.

CORONARY ARTERY BYPASS GRAFT SURGERY AND STROKE

Atherosclerosis of the ascending aorta may be a more important cause of perioperative stroke than carotid artery stenosis.[90]

Carotid Stenosis

The rate of stroke is elevated in patients with carotid stenosis who have CABG. The available data suggests that unilateral asymptomatic carotid stenosis of 50-99% is not an independent risk factor for ipsilateral ischemic stroke with CABG. In contrast, certain groups of patients with carotid artery disease appear to have an increased risk of stroke with CABG, including the following:[91]

- Symptomatic carotid stenosis of 50-99% in men and 70-99% in women
- Bilateral asymptomatic stenosis of 80-99%
- Unilateral asymptomatic stenosis of 70-99% and contralateral carotid occlusion.

Thus, prophylactic carotid revascularization is only recommended in these patients. Prophylactic revascularization of unilateral asymptomatic significant carotid stenosis is not recommended prior to CABG surgery.

Carotid Endarterectomy versus Carotid Stenting

In the situations requiring urgent CABG like ACS or left main coronary disease simultaneous carotid endarterectomy (CEA) and CABG surgery is preferred, if carotid revascularization is also indicated.

In patients in whom CABG surgery is not urgent and needs carotid revascularization, CEA or carotid artery stenting (CAS) may be done prophylactically. If CAS is done, CABG surgery is deferred for a few weeks, as it mandates dual antiplatelet treatment initially, which can increase intraoperative bleeding.

Irrespective of treatment strategy, aggressive medical treatment including statins and antiplatelets is the cornerstone in the management of combined carotid and coronary disease.

Timing of Coronary Artery Bypass Graft Surgery after Stroke

Prior history of stroke or TIA predisposes to increased risk of perioperative stroke after CABG surgery. So unless the CABG surgery is urgent, it is deferred for several weeks after cerebral ischemic event. The optimal timing of CABG surgery depends upon multiple factors, including the size of the stroke, the risk of stroke recurrence (which is, in turn, dependent on the stroke mechanism), and the urgency of cardiac intervention. The delay ensures for post-stroke recovery of autoregulatory capabilities of the cerebral vasculature prior to exposure to periprocedural hypotension, and for sufficient remodeling of the damaged parenchyma to decrease the risk of hemorrhagic transformation of the infarct.

Epilogue

Simultaneous or sequential occurrence of myocardial infarction and stroke poses complex and challenging scenario to the treating team of cardiologist and neurologist. This is due to their life-threatening nature, narrow but different window period of treatment. The therapeutic modalities for treatment of both involve mechanical intervention, thrombolysis, anticoagulation and antiplatelet administration. However, it is the timing of specific treatment, which decides whether either or both organ systems benefit or have disastrous consequences.

Thrombolysis for STEMI is absolutely contraindicated with any prior intracranial hemorrhage or ischemic stroke within last 3 months.

- STEMI with ischemic stroke less than 3 hours:
  - Ideally mechanical thrombectomy for stroke and primary PCI for MI at the same sitting, if feasible and if not
  - Thrombolysis for stroke, if patient is hemodynamically stable and PCI later (after 24 hours when DAPT is permitted), if unstable primary PCI and conservative management of stroke

- STEMI with more than 1 month old prior stroke:
  - Primary PCI (as 75% of hemorrhagic stroke conversion occurs in 4 days and rest in 3 weeks)
- STEMI with ischemic stroke more than 3 hours old and less than 1 month:
  - Individualized strategy depending upon chances of hemorrhagic conversion:
    - A small lacunar infarct more than 4 days old with low chances of hemorrhagic transformation: Primary PCI
    - If significant chances of hemorrhagic conversion, thrombus aspiration only or use of bare metal stent to avoid aggressive DAPT regime.
- STEMI with intracranial hemorrhage:
  - Since chances of hematoma expansion after 24 hours are low, if hemodynamic condition demands, primary PCI may be undertaken, especially if ICH score is low. Here, intraprocedural single dose of heparin may not be too risky but aggressive antiplatelet regimen as far as possible needs to be avoided
- CABG surgery after stroke: If not urgent, it should be delayed for several weeks till cerebral autoregulation recovers and cerebral parenchyma remodeling is complete
- Prophylactic intervention before CABG surgery of asymptomatic unilateral carotid stenosis is not recommended even when severe.

REFERENCES

1. Chin PL, Kaminski J, Rout M. Myocardial infarction coincident with cerebrovascular accidents in the elderly. Age Ageing. 1977;6:29-37.
2. Caplan LR. Brain embolism, revisited. Neurology. 1993;43:1281-7.
3. Bentzon JF, Otsuka F, Virmani R, et al. Mechanisms of plaque formation and rupture. Circ Res. 2014;114:1852-66.
4. Pinero P, Gonzalez A, Martinez E, et al. Volume and composition of emboli in neuroprotected stenting of the carotid artery. Am J Neuroradiol. 2009;30:473-8.
5. Sadowski M, Zabczyk M, Undas A. Coronary thrombus composition: links with inflammation, platelet and endothelial markers. Atherosclerosis. 2014;237:555-61.
6. Fabbri D, Long Q, Das S, et al. Computational modelling of emboli travel trajectories in cerebral arteries: influence of microembolic particle size and density. Biomech Model Mechanobiol. 2014;13:289-302.
7. Cipolla MJ. The cerebral circulation. Colloquium series in integrated systems physiology: form molecule to function. Milton Keyes: Morgan & Claypool Life Sciences; 2010.
8. Schoknecht K, David Y, Heinemann U. The blood-brain barrier-Gatekeeper to neuronal homeostasis: Clinical implications in the setting of stroke. Semin Cell Dev Biol. 2015;38:35-42.
9. Camici PG, d'Amati G, Rimoldi O. Coronary microvascular dysfunction: mechanisms and functional assessment. Nat Rev Cardiol. 2015;12:48-62.
10. Schaper W, Schaper J. Collateral Circulation: Heart, Brain, Kidney, Limbs. Boston: Kluwer Academic Publishers; 1993.
11. Sheth SA, Liebeskind DS. Imaging evaluation of collaterals in the brain: physiology and clinical translation. Curr Radiol Rep. 2014;2:29.
12. Blinder P, Tsai PS, Kaufhold JP, et al. The cortical angiome: an interconnected vascular network with noncolumnar patterns of blood flow. Nat Neurosci. 2013;16:889-97.

13. Zimarino M, D'Andreamatteo M, Waksman R, et al. The dynamics of the coronary collateral circulation. Nat Rev Cardiol. 2014;11:191-7.
14. Norving B. Oxford Textbook of Stroke and Cerebrovascular Disease. Oxford: Oxford University Press; 2014.
15. Zinkstok SM, Roos YB. Early administration of aspirin in patients treated with alteplase for acute ischaemic stroke: A randomised controlled trial. Lancet. 2012;380:731-7.
16. Sandercock PA, Counsell C, Kane EJ. Anticoagulants for acute ischaemic stroke. Cochrane Database Syst Rev. 2015;3:CD000024.
17. Jauch EC, Saver JL, Adams HP Jr, et al. Guidelines for the early management of patients with acute ischemic stroke: a guideline for healthcare professionals from the American Heart Association/American Stroke Association. Stroke. 2013;44:870-947.
18. Omar HR, Fathy A, Rashad R, et al. Concomitant acute right ventricular infarction and ischemic cerebrovascular stroke: possible explanations. Int Arch Med. 2010;3:25.
19. Yeo LL, Andersson T, Yee KW, et al. Synchronous cardiocerebral infarction in the era of endovascular therapy: which to treat first? J Thromb Thrombolysis. 2017;44:104-11.
20. Gunnoo T, Hasan N, Khan MS, et al. Quantifying the risk of heart disease following acute ischaemic stroke: a meta-analysis of over 50,000 participants. BMJ Open. 2016;6:e009535.
21. Witt BJ, Ballman KV, Brown RD, et al. The incidence of stroke after myocardial infarction: a meta-analysis. Am J Med. 2006;119:354.e1-9.
22. Gattringer T, Niederkorn K, Seyfang L, et al. Myocardial infarction as a complication in acute stroke: results from the Austrian Stroke Unit Registry. Cerebrovasc Dis. 2014;37:147-52.
23. Saczynski JS, Spencer FA, Gore JM, et al. Twenty-year trends in the incidence of stroke complicating acute myocardial infarction: Worcester heart attack study. Arch Intern Med. 2008;168:2104-10.
24. Budaj A, Flasinska K, Gore JM, et al. Magnitude of and risk factors for in-hospital and post-discharge stroke in patients with acute coronary syndromes: findings from a Global Registry of Acute Coronary Events. Circulation. 2005;111:3242-7.
25. Tokuda K, Shindo S, Yamada K, et al. Acute embolic cerebral infarction and coronary artery embolism in a patient with atrial fibrillation caused by similar thrombi. J Stroke Cerebrovasc Dis. 2016;25:1797-9.
26. Kim HL, Seo JB, Chung WY, et al. Simultaneously presented acute ischemic stroke and non-ST elevation myocardial infarction in a patient with paroxysmal atrial fibrillation. Korean Circ J. 2013;43:766-9.
27. Nguyen TL, Rajaratnam R. Dissecting out the cause: a case of concurrent acute myocardial infarction and stroke. BMJ Case Rep. 2011;2011:pii: bcr0220113824.
28. Verma GC, Jain G, Wahid A, et al. Acute ischaemic stroke and acute myocardial infarction occurring together in domestic low-voltage (220-240V) electrical injury: a rare complication. J Assoc Physicians India. 2014;62:620-3.
29. Nagai M, Hoshide S, Kario K. The insular cortex and cardiovascular system: a new insight into the brain-heart axis. J Am Soc Hypertens. 2010;4:174-82.
30. Ay H, Koroshetz WJ, Benner T, et al. Neuroanatomic correlates of stroke-related myocardial injury. Neurology. 2006;66:1325-9.
31. O'Gara PT, Kushner FG, Ascheim DD, et al. 2013 ACCF/AHA Guideline for the management of ST-elevation myocardial infarction: a report of the American College of Cardiology Foundation/American Heart Association Task Force on Practice Guidelines. Circulation. 2013;127:e362-425.
32. Amsterdam EA, Wenger NK, Brindis RG, et al. 2014 AHA/ACC Guideline for the management of patients with non–ST-elevation acute coronary syndromes. Circulation. 2014; 130:e344.
33. Demaerschalk BM, Kleindorfer DO, Adeoye OM, et al. Scientific rationale for the inclusion and exclusion criteria for intravenous alteplase in acute ischemic stroke: a

statement for healthcare professionals from the American Heart Association/American Stroke Association. Stroke. 2016;47:581-641.
34. Goyal M, Menon BK, van Zwam WH, et al. Endovascular thrombectomy after large-vessel ischaemic stroke: a meta-analysis of individual patient data from five randomised trials. Lancet. 2016;387:1723-31.
35. Hanne L, Brunecker P, Grittner U, et al. Right insular infarction and mortality after ischaemic stroke. Eur J Neurol. 2017;24:67-72.
36. Sposato LA, Cohen G, Wardlaw JM, et al. Effect of right insular involvement on death and functional outcome after acute ischemic stroke in the IST-3 trial (Third International Stroke Trial). Stroke. 2016;47:2959-65.
37. Goldberg RJ, Steg PG, Sadiq I, et al. Extent of, and factors associated with, delay to hospital presentation in patients with acute coronary disease (the GRACE registry). Am J Cardiol. 2002;89:791-6.
38. Skolnick AH, Alexander KP, Chen AY, et al. Characteristics, management, and outcomes of 5,557 patients age > or = 90 years with acute coronary syndromes: results from the CRUSADE Initiative. J Am Coll Cardiol. 2007;49:1790-7.
39. Devlin G, Gore JM, Elliott J, et al. Management and 6-month outcomes in elderly and very elderly patients with high-risk non-ST elevation acute coronary syndromes: the Global Registry of Acute Coronary Events. Eur Heart J. 2008;29:1275-82.
40. White HD. Thrombolytic therapy in the elderly. Lancet. 2000;356:2028-30.
41. Zhang M, Guddeti RR, Wang SP, et al. Prior ischemic stroke is not associated with worse clinical outcomes in patients undergoing percutaneous coronary intervention. Clin Invest Med. 2014;37(4): E196-202.
42. Myint PK, Kwok CS, Roffe C, et al. Determinants and Outcomes of Stroke Following Percutaneous Coronary Intervention by Indication. Stroke. 2016;47(6):1500-7.
43. Werner N, Zeymer U. Stroke outcomes in patients undergoing percutaneous coronary intervention in clinical practice today. Interv Cardiol. 2011;3(3):407-13.
44. Cale L, Constantino R. Strategies for decreasing vascular complications in diagnostic cardiac catheterization patients. Dimens Crit Care Nurs. 2012;31(1):13-7.
45. Harmon M, Baron JC, Viader F, et al. Periprocedural stroke and cardiac catheterization. Circulation. 2008;118:678-83.
46. Segal AZ, Abernethy WB, Palacios IF, et al. Stroke as a complication of cardiac catheterization: Risk factors and clinical features. Neurology. 2001;56:975-6.
47. Zhang H, Feng LQ, Qang YP. Characteristics and risk factors of cerebrovascular accidents after percutaneous coronary interventions in patients with history of stroke. Chin Med J. 2010;123(12):1515-9.
48. Sankaranarayanan R, Msairi A, Davis GK. Stroke complicating cardiac catheterization—A preventable and treatable complication. J Invasive Cardiol. 2007;19(1):40-5.
49. Khatri P, Kasner SE. Ischemic strokes after cardiac catheterization: Opportune thrombolysis candidates? Arch Neurol. 2006;63(6):817-21.
50. Lin CF, Chu KC, Wang M. Acute ischemic stroke after percutaneous cardiac intervention in an elderly patient. Int J Gerontol. 2012;4(1):43-6.
51. Duffis EJ, Jones D, Tighe D, et al. Neurological complications of coronary angiographic procedures. Exp Rev Cardiovasc Ther. 2007;5(6):1113-21.
52. McPherson TP, Dighe K, Charania J, et al. (2012). Cardiac catheterization and periprocedural stroke. CCC 2012 Abstract. [online] Available from http://www.pulsus.com/ccc2010/abs/546.htm. [Last accessed May, 2019].
53. Hoffman SJ, Routledge HC, Lennon RJ, et al. Procedural factors associated with percutaneous coronary intervention-related ischemic stroke. J Am Coll Cardiol Intv. 2012;5:200-6.
54. Zeus T, Ketterer U, Leuf D, et al. Safety of percutaneous coronary intervention in patients with acute ischemic stroke/transient ischemic attack and acute coronary syndrome. Clin Res Cardiol. 2016;105(4):356-63.

55. Guptill JT, Mehta RH, Armstrong PW, et al. Stroke after primary percutaneous coronary intervention in patients with ST-segment elevation myocardial infarction timing, characteristics, and clinical outcomes. Circ Cardiovasc Interv. 2013;6(2):176-83.
56. Tamhane UU, Chetcuti S, Hameed I, et al. Safety and efficacy of thrombectomy in patients undergoing primary percutaneous coronary intervention for acute ST elevation MI: a meta-analysis of randomized controlled trials. BMC Cardiovasc Disord. 2010;10:10.
57. Tanne D, Gottlieb S, Hod H, et al. Incidence and mortality from early stroke associated myocardial infarction in the prethrombolytic and thrombolytic eras. Secondary Prevention Reinfarction Israeli Nifedipine Trial (SPRINT) and Israeli Thrombolytic Survey Groups. J Am Coll Cardiol. 1997;30:1484-90.
58. Cronin L, Mehta SR, Zhao F, et al. Stroke in relation to cardiac procedures in patients with non-ST-elevation acute coronary syndrome: a study involving >18,000 patients. Circulation. 2001;104:269-74.
59. Mooe T, Olofsson BO, Stegmayr B. Ischemic stroke: impact of a recent myocardial infarction. Stroke. 1999;30:997-1001.
60. Witt BJ, Brown RD, Jacobson SJ, et al. A community-based study of stroke incidence after myocardial infarction. Ann Intern Med. 2005;143:785-92.
61. American Heart Association. (2005). Heart disease and stroke statistics—2005 update. [online] Available from www.americanheart.org. [Last accessed May, 2019].
62. Fibrinolytic Therapy Trialists' Collaborative Group. Indications for fibrinolytic therapy in suspected acute myocardial infarction: collaborative overview of early mortality and major morbidity results from all randomized trials of more than 1000 patients. Lancet. 1994;343:311-22.
63. Wienbergen H, Schiele R, Gitt AK, et al. Incidence, risk factors, and clinical outcome of stroke after acute myocardial infarction in clinical practice. Am J Cardiol. 2001;87:782-5.
64. Kassem-Moussa H, Mahaffey KW, Graffagnino C, et al. Incidence and characteristics of stroke during 90-day follow-up in patients stabilized after an acute coronary syndrome. Am Heart J. 2004;148:439-46.
65. Lichtman JH, Krumholz HM, Wang Y, et al. Risks and predictors of stroke after myocardial infarction among the elderly. Results from the co-operative cardiovascular project. Circulation. 2002;105:1082-7.
66. Mooe T, Eriksson P, Stegmayr B. Ischemic stroke after acute myocardial infarction. A population-based study. Stroke. 1997;28:762-7.
67. Vaitkus PT, Barnathan ES. Embolic potential, prevention, and management of mural thrombus complicating anterior myocardial infarction: a meta-analysis. J Am Coll Cardiol. 1993;22:1004-9.
68. Greaves SC, Zhi G, Lee RT, et al. Incidence and natural history of left ventricular thrombus following anterior wall acute myocardial infarction. Am J Cardiol. 1997;80:442-8.
69. Merlini PA, Bauer KA, Oltrona L, et al. Persistent activation of coagulation mechanism in unstable angina and myocardial infarction. Circulation. 1994;90:61-8.
70. Lombardo A, Biasucci LM, Lanza GA, et al. Inflammation as a possible link between coronary and carotid plaque instability. Circulation. 2004;109:3158-63.
71. Mahaffey KW, Granger CB, Sloan MA, et al. Risk factors for in-hospital nonhemorrhagic stroke in patients with acute myocardial infarction treated with thrombolysis. Results from GUSTO-1. Circulation. 1998;97:757-64.
72. Yusuf S, Flather M, Pogue J, et al. Variations between countries in invasive cardiac procedures and outcomes in patients with suspected unstable angina or myocardial infarction without initial ST elevation. OASIS Registry investigators. Lancet. 1998;352:507-14.
73. Pfeiffer MA, McMurray JJ, Velazquez EJ, et al. Valsartan, Captopril or both in myocardial infarction complicated by heart failure, left ventricular dysfunction or both. N Engl J Med. 2003;349:1893-906.

74. The CURE Investigators. Effects of clopidogrel in addition to aspirin in patients with acute coronary syndromes without ST-segment elevation. N Engl J Med. 2001;345:494-502.
75. CAPRIE Steering Committee. A randomised, blinded trial of clopidogrel versus aspirin in patients at risk of ischaemic events. Lancet. 1996;348:1329-39.
76. Theroux P, Waters D, Lam J, et al. Reactivation of unstable angina after the discontinuation of heparin. N Engl J Med. 1992;372:141-5.
77. van Es RF, Jonker JJ, Verheught FW, et al. Aspirin and coumadin after acute coronary syndromes: a randomized controlled trial. Lancet. 2002;360:109-13.
78. Hurlen M, Abdelnoor M, Smith P, et al. Warfarin, aspirin, or both after myocardial infarction. N Engl J Med. 2002;347:969-74.
79. CARS Investigators. Randomized double-blind trial of fixed low-dose warfarin with aspirin after myocardial infarction. Lancet. 1997;350:389-96.
80. Fiore LD, Ezekowitz MD, Brophy MT, et al. Department of Veterans Affairs Cooperative Studies Program clinical trial comparing combined warfarin and aspirin with aspirin alone in survivors of acute myocardial infarction: primary results of the CHAMP study. Circulation. 2002;105:557-63.
81. Herlitz J, Holm J, Peterson M, et al. Factors associated with development of stroke long-term after myocardial infarction: experiences from the LoWASA trial. J Intern Med. 2005;257:201-7.
82. Deliargyris EN, Upadhya B, Applegate RJ, et al. Safety of abciximab administration during PCI of patients with previous stroke. J Thromb Thrombolysis. 2005;19(3):147-53.
83. Serebruany VL. Viewpoint: paradoxical excess mortality in the PLATO trial should be independently verified. Thromb Haemost. 2011;105:752-9.
84. US Food and Drug Administration. (2011). The FDA ticagrelor review of complete response. [online] Available from http://www.accessdata.fda.gov/drugsatfda_docs/nda/2011/022433Orig1s000TOC.cfm. [Last accessed May, 2019].
85. Fujii Y, Tanaka R, Takeuchi S, et al. Hematoma enlargement in spontaneous intracerebral haemorrhage. J Neurosurgery. 1994;80:51-7.
86. Paciaroni M, Agnelli G, Venti M, et al. Efficacy and safety of anticoagulants in the prevention of venous thromboembolism in patients with acute cerebral hemorrhage: a meta-analysis of controlled studies. J Thromb Haemost. 2011;9:893-8.
87. McQuaid KR, Laine L. Systematic review and meta-analysis of adverse events of low-dose aspirin and clopidogrel in randomized controlled trials. Am J Med. 2006;119:624-38.
88. Ding X, Liu X, Tan C, et al. Resumption of antiplatelet therapy in patients with primary intracranial hemorrhage-benefits and risks: A meta-analysis of cohort studies. J Neurol Sci. 2018;384:133-8.
89. Hemphill JC 3rd, Bonovich DC, Besmertis L, et al. The ICH score: a simple, reliable grading scale for intracerebral hemorrhage. Stroke. 2001;32:891-7.
90. Yeh RW, Secemsky E, Kereiakes DJ, et al. Development and validation of a prediction rule for benefit and harm of dual antiplatelet therapy beyond one year after percutaneous coronary intervention: an analysis from the randomized Dual Antiplatelet Therapy Study. JAMA. March 2016.
91. Naylor AR, Bown MJ. Stroke after cardiac surgery and its association with asymptomatic carotid disease: an updated systematic review and meta-analysis. Eur J Vasc Endovasc Surg. 2011;41:607-24.

CHAPTER 3

Acute Coronary Syndrome with Chronic Kidney Disease

> **Prologue**
> **A Tale of Two Teachers**
> A few years ago, one of my teachers got admitted due to acute left ventricular failure (LVF). He was long-standing diabetic and had serum creatinine of 1.9 mg%. In view of left ventricular dysfunction and electrocardiography (ECG) changes, his coronary angiogram was done by taking due precautions needed to prevent contrast-induced nephropathy (CIN). He had a critical lesion in proximal right coronary angiogram, which the author stented in the same sitting. A total of around 30 mL of nonionic contrast was used. Hemodynamically he settled; however, his creatinine started rising and ultimately ended up needing regular dialysis for next few years. During this period, cardiologically he was stable and never had any further cardiac-related symptoms or hospitalization. However my teacher and his relatives who did not overtly express, the author know attributed this to the angiogram and angioplasty.
>
> A few days later, another of my teachers with long-standing diabetes with baseline creatinine of 2.3 mg% presented with acute LVF due to acute coronary syndrome (ACS). Getting wiser from earlier experience, the author explained the inherent risk of progression of renal failure and took him for coronary angiogram, which too showed a critical proximal right coronary artery (RCA) lesion which the author stented consuming a maximum of 30 mL of contrast. He too got stabilized and was cardiac-wise asymptomatic for more than 3 years with creatinine hovering around 2.5 mg%. He is dialysis free till date.

■ INTRODUCTION

During the past decade, chronic kidney disease (CKD) has emerged as an important prognostic marker for mortality and morbidity after myocardial infarction (MI). Even a mild derangement of kidney function affects prognosis in acute coronary syndrome (ACS).[1] Reduction of as little as 10 mL of estimated glomerular filtration rate (eGFR), after 70–90 mL/min, increases the rate of mortality by 10–14% after an episode of MI. As kidney function declines, mortality increases in both symptomatic and asymptomatic heart disease patients. Since majority of the patients with ST segment elevation myocardial infarction (STEMI) are subjected to percutaneous coronary intervention (PCI) involving potentially nephrotoxic contrast agents, it is prudent that the treating physicians must be aware of the association between kidney disease and coronary artery disease (CAD).

■ EPIDEMIOLOGY

Many epidemiological studies have revealed a distinct relationship between cardiovascular events and kidney disease. GFR is an independent risk factor for various cardiovascular events including peripheral arterial disease (PAD), CAD and heart failure as reported in a systematic review of 1.4 million adults from 42 different cohorts.[2] According to this review, the risk of all-cause mortality was highest in patients with the lowest baseline GFR. In view of the mounting evidence through epidemiological studies, the American College of Cardiology/American Heart Association (ACC/AHA) and the National Kidney Foundation (NKF) recommend that CKD should be considered as equivalent to CAD for the risk of mortality and morbidity.

■ PATHOPHYSIOLOGY OF CAD IN CKD

Atherosclerosis is a condition characterized by formation of calcific plaques in the intimal layers of vessels. In CAD, in general population, atherosclerotic plaques in the intimal layers are responsible for majority of the cardiovascular events. However, pathophysiological mechanisms of vascular disease in kidney disease are different. Apart from the known risk factors such as hypertension, diabetes and dyslipidemia, endothelial dysfunction (ED), CKD-MBD (CKD–mineral and bone disorder) abnormalities, increased oxidative stress and local inflammation are likely to play an important role in the vascular disease in patients with CKD and end-stage renal disease (ESRD) when compared to healthy subjects.[3] Several studies have demonstrated that persistent systemic inflammation may be responsible for the increased risk in patients with ESRD irrespective of renal replacement therapy.[3] Biomarkers such as C-reactive protein, interleukin and tumor necrosis factor (TNF) are seen to be deranged in cardiovascular disease (CVD) and CKD populations.[3] Nonetheless, the reasons for worse cardiovascular outcomes in patients with CKD are still unclear.

It is hypothesized by Charytan et al. that unlike the general population, the patients with CKD may fail to develop collateral circulation to overcome obstructive CAD.[4] This finding may explain worse cardiovascular outcome in patients with CKD. However, their own study showed that patients with CKD and without CKD had a similar culprit artery collateral supply disproving their own hypothesis.[4] In this context, the role of vascular calcification in the vessel wall assumes greater significance. There is a close relationship between vascular calcification and mortality due to CAD, particularly in patients with kidney disease. Calcification in the intimal layers and tunica media, known as Monckeberg's sclerosis, is more common in patients with CKD compared to general population.[5] The calcification in the vessel wall, particularly the medial layer, leads to decrease in coronary microcirculation and arterial elasticity resulting in adverse hemodynamics.

Complex interaction between increased levels of proinflammatory cytokines, malnutrition and atherosclerosis/calcification in patients with end-stage kidney disease is described as MIAC (malnutrition, inflammation, atherosclerosis, calcification) syndrome. This syndrome is frequently associated with increased mortality and morbidity in patients receiving peritoneal dialysis (PD) as well as hemodialysis (HD).[6] A recent study elegantly demonstrated a significant correlation between increased coronary artery calcification score (CACS) and decreased coronary flow velocity reserve (CFR) in patients undergoing HD.[7]

Epicardial adipose tissue (EAT), which is true visceral fat, is yet another significant determinant of severity of CAD in patients with CKD. Although its precise role in CAD is not yet clear, it is hypothesized that EAT may stimulate production of proinflammatory and proatherogenic cytokines leading to obstructive CAD in patients with end-stage kidney disease.[8]

■ CKD AS AN INDEPENDENT RISK FACTOR FOR CAD

Reduction in GFR as well as proteinuria increases the risk for CVD. The relationship between kidney disease and heightened risk for CVD is demonstrated in community-based population as well as in general population at high risk for CVD. Community-based populations include cohorts that were not specifically selected to enroll patients with CKD or CVD. On the contrary, the general population studies include cohorts with specific recruitment of patients with either pre-existing CVD or patients with heightened risk factors for CAD.

■ ASSOCIATION BETWEEN CKD AND CAD IN COMMUNITY-BASED POPULATION

A meta-analysis of general population cohorts[9] perhaps provides reliable data regarding association between CKD and heart disease. This study included 105,872 participants with measurements of urine albumin to creatinine ratio (ACR) and 1,128,310 participants with dipstick measurements of urine protein. The baseline levels of eGFR were available for all the participants of this study. This study estimated the hazard ratios (HRs) for all-cause mortality during a follow-up period of 7.9 years. The study compared the all-cause mortality among patients with a baseline eGFR of 95 mL/min/1.73 m^2 with those patients with reduced GFRs of 60, 45, and 15 mL/min/1.73 m^2. The study found that HRs for all-cause mortality as well cardiovascular mortality increased as the GFR decreased. In this, proteinuria was independently associated with increase in all-cause and cardiovascular mortality.[9] The study also found that as the urine ACR increased, the HR for all-cause mortality and cardiovascular mortality also increased correspondingly.

Framingham risk score, which is a well-known and a traditional method to analyze and predict future cardiovascular events, does not consider renal parameters of the participants. Since CKD alone apparently increases risk for heart disease, it is to be expected that Framingham cohort study provides poor overall accuracy in predicting CVD in patients with CKD. It is also to be expected that inclusion of ACR and estimated GFR along with traditional cardiovascular risk factors increases the ability to forecast cardiovascular events.

ASSOCIATION BETWEEN CKD AND CHD AMONG THOSE AT HIGH CARDIOVASCULAR RISK

Many secondary analyses of studies have shown that various degree of renal dysfunction is independently associated with cardiovascular events.[10,11] These studies have enrolled patients with known risk factors for coronary heart disease (CHD) such as hypertension and diabetes or pre-existing heart disease. A collaborative meta-analysis of 10 cohorts consisting of 266,975 patients[11] with hypertension, diabetes, CVD, or a combination of these factors amply demonstrates the magnitude of association between renal function, proteinuria and cardiovascular outcomes. A monotonic association between high ACR and heightened risk for cardiovascular and all-cause mortality was also noted in this study.

CKD AS A CHD RISK EQUIVALENT

The concept of "risk equivalence" for heart disease was developed by many expert panels to guide the treating physicians regarding how aggressive they can be in their treatment to prevent heart disease in their patients. In view of a significant body of evidence in favor of association between mild-to-moderate CKD and CVD, ACC/AHA and NKF recommended in their older guidelines that CKD may be considered as a risk equivalent to CHD.[12] Diabetes too is considered a risk equivalent for CHD. In the studies conducted by Alberta Kidney Disease Network and Atherosclerosis Risk in Communities (ARIC), the number of cardiovascular events attributable to CKD was similar to the events attributable to diabetes.[13] However, many recent expert panels have moved away from the concept of risk equivalence and instead suggested recommendations for preventive therapies based on 10-year risk for heart disease. The generalization that CKD is a CHD "risk equivalent" for all patients with CKD is unwarranted for the following reasons:

- Some studies contradict the concept of CKD as a CHD risk equivalent. For instance, in a study conducted by Alberta Kidney Disease Network, the 4-year incidence of MI was almost 3-fold higher among patients who had a prior history of MI (7.7%) compared to those patients who had a prior history of MI and CKD (2.8%).[13] In this study, incidence of MI in patients with no prior history of MI but no prior history of diabetes or CKD was two-times more than those with prior history of diabetes or CKD but no prior history of MI. Similarly, an ARIC study revealed that risk associated with CKD was not comparable to the risk accompanying prior history of MI[14]
- The risk of heart disease in those with CKD apparently varies based upon absolute levels of renal function and degree of protein loss in the urine. In addition, the risk varies depending on the rate at which various renal factors change
- The patients with certain degree of renal dysfunction may not have same level of risk for CHD because risk for CVD in a patient with CKD is in part related to other comorbidities. For instance, the overall risk for a 25-year-old nonsmoker with CKD due to IgA nephropathy is different from the risk posed to a 65-year-old man with a similar degree of CKD with history of chronic smoking, hypertension and hypercholesterolemia.

TRADITIONAL AND NONTRADITIONAL CARDIOVASCULAR RISK FACTORS IN CKD

Traditional risk factors of heart disease such as hypertension, smoking, diabetes, dyslipidemia and old age are frequently associated with CKD populations as well.[12,15] Moreover, the frequency of cardiovascular risk factors appears to correlate with severity of derangement of renal function.[15] The metabolic syndrome consisting of insulin resistance, dyslipidemia, elevated serum levels of glucose, abdominal obesity and hypertension is more frequently associated with CKD. This metabolic syndrome contributes to the increased risk for CVD.

Nontraditional risk factors for heart disease but unique to patients with CKD include retention of uremic toxins, anemia, increased serum levels of certain cytokines, abnormalities of bone mineral metabolism and/or an "increased inflammatory-poor nutrition state".[16] Disorders of bone mineral metabolism in CKD are increasingly associated with coronary artery calcification.

REDUCTION OF CHD RISK IN PATIENTS WITH CKD

It is now well-established that in patients with no kidney disease, risk factor modification and beneficial lifestyle changes can substantially decrease morbidity and mortality in patients with CAD, cerebrovascular disease, and

PAD. However, since most of the clinical trials involving CAD in the past have excluded patients with kidney disease, preventive guidelines in this context are scanty. However, randomized trials have subsequently been performed in patients with CKD—with particular reference to statin therapy. Since many studies conclude that CKD is not an equivalent risk as CHD, the ideal guidelines for prevention of heart disease in CKD populations should be based on available data and future cardiovascular risk.

■ STATIN THERAPY

Most evidence for the use of statins in patients with mild-to-moderate CKD comes from post-hoc subgroup analyses of randomized trials that were not intended to include patients with deranged renal function. The SHARP trial evaluated lowering of cholesterol levels with statins to prevent heart disease in patients with CKD.[17] This trial concluded that use of statins in patient with CKD not requiring dialysis significantly reduces the risk for adverse cardiovascular events. However, since these studies predominantly included older patients, it is not clear whether statin therapy as a preventive measure would be effective in younger patients with a primary kidney disease such as IgA nephropathy or ADPKD. Nonetheless, it would be desirable to provide statin therapy in patients with an eGFR less than 60 mL/min/1.73 m^2.

■ BLOOD PRESSURE CONTROL

Post-hoc analyses of CKD subgroups from cardiovascular trials conclude that treatment with antihypertensive drugs reduces the risk of major cardiovascular events.[18-20] However, in patients with kidney disease, especially nonproteinuric CKD, no specific antihypertensive drug is found to provide preferential cardiovascular benefit. A meta-analysis examined cardiovascular outcomes and mortality in 30,295 patients enrolled for 26 randomized hypertension trials.[19] These patients had a GFR of less than 60 mL/min/1.73 m^2 and 93% of these patients were nonproteinuric. Follow-up of these patients for a period of 4 years revealed the following findings:
- Compared to placebo, angiotensin-converting enzyme (ACE) inhibitors and calcium channel antagonists reduced incidence of cardiovascular events and mortality. Trials comparing β-blockers and diuretics with placebo were excluded in this meta-analysis
- In drug versus drug trials, incidence of cardiovascular events and mortality were similar comparing angiotensin inhibitors with diuretics or β-blockers or with calcium channel antagonists.

However, in patients with proteinuria (defined as 500–1,000 mg/day), there is evidence that ACE inhibitors provide some benefit when compared to patients with nonproteinuric CKD. In such cases, ACE inhibitors are known to reduce progression of renal disease.

ANTIPLATELET THERAPY

It is known that long-term therapy with aspirin reduces the risk of subsequent MI, stroke and vascular death in patients with no proven kidney disease. However, there is inadequate data regarding efficacy as well as safety of antiplatelet therapy in patients with kidney disease. A meta-analysis of 27,139 patients with CKD was done to test the effectiveness of aspirin and other antiplatelet agents to prevent heart disease.[21] This meta-analysis concluded that antiplatelet therapy significantly reduces the incidence of fatal and nonfatal MI as compared to placebo or no therapy. However, aspirin therapy also increased the rate of major bleeding in patients with CKD. Based on the findings of these trials, it is prudent that decision regarding use of antiplatelet drugs to prevent heart disease in patients with CKD must be individualized and it must depend on the patient's overall risk for CHD and major bleeding. The prescription of low-dose aspirin is reasonably safe in most patients with CKD.

TREATMENT OF CHD IN PATIENTS WITH CKD

Patients with CKD are prone to drug-related adverse effects. Hence, they require scrupulous attention to dosage of drugs. However, despite the increased risk of side effects, the treatment strategies such as revascularization to treat established heart disease in patients with no kidney disease are known to be equally effective in patients with CKD.[22] Many studies have shown that medical therapy used in patients without kidney disease is less frequently used in patients with kidney disease. A study consisting of 889 patients with ACS with kidney disease (GFR of less than 60 mL/min/1.73 m^2) showed that patients with renal dysfunction were less likely to receive PCI[23] and reduced usage of glycoprotein (GP) IIb/IIIa inhibitor.

However, not all the usual treatment methods used in patients without kidney disease should be universally employed in patients with CKD. It has been reported that use of GP IIb/IIIa inhibitor or clopidogrel increased the risk of major bleeding episodes without any significant cardiovascular benefit.[21]

PROGNOSIS OF CHD IN PATIENTS WITH CKD

A common finding in patients who undergo intervention for cardiac events is that they have worse prognosis, if there is a concurrent renal dysfunction. However, underlying mechanisms for worse prognosis are not clear. One of the probable reasons for worse prognosis is that patients with kidney disease and who suffer a cardiac event have other usual predictors of adverse outcomes such as old age, hypotension and low body weight. Another possibility is that adverse outcome attributed to renal dysfunction may instead suggest a more severe form of ACS.

ACUTE MYOCARDIAL INFARCTION WITH ACUTE KIDNEY INJURY

Acute kidney injury (AKI), known earlier as acute renal failure, occurs frequently in many patients hospitalized for various ailments. In post-MI setting, AKI has an independent association with long-term mortality. As little as 0.1 mg/dL increase in serum creatinine is known to increase the risk of ESRD and all-cause mortality in post-MI setting.[24] AKI is particularly common after cardiac surgery and associated with increased risk of death.[25]

The long-term implications of AKI are well documented. However, the trials on risk of early AKI in post-MI setting are not many. A trial by Fox et al. including a large number of patients (n = 59,970) drawn from ACTION registry has attempted to document risk of AKI in post-MI setting.[26]

This study found that overall prevalence of AKI in the setting of MI is 16%. Patients with AKI in this trial had a significant risk of mortality when compared to those without AKI. In addition, these patients had a heightened risk of in-hospital major bleeding events. The risk of AKI is as high as 24% after cardiac surgery and as many as 1.1% of them require dialysis. When acute myocardial infarction (AMI) is complicated by cardiogenic shock, the AKI may afflict almost half the number of patients.[26]

Evidence for short-term mortality in the setting of post-MI setting and AKI is scanty. In a single-center study in Israel consisting of 1,038 patients who presented with STEMI, an 11.4-fold increased risk of in-hospital mortality was associated with worsening renal function.[27] Substantial short-term increased risks of AKI have been observed outside of AMI setting. For instance, among 27,068 patients who underwent coronary angiography (CAG) over a 12-year period, small changes in serum creatinine (0.25–0.50 mg/dL) were associated with 1.83-fold increased risk of mortality, while patients with more than 1.0 mg/dL increase in serum creatinine was associated with 3-fold increased risk of mortality.[28]

Complications associated with AKI are particularly pronounced after cardiac surgery. A recent multicenter cohort study found that participants with as little as 25% decrease in eGFR had a 4-fold increased risk of postoperative mortality. In this study, postoperative mortality increased by 9.5-fold when eGFR fell by 75%.[25] There is ample evidence in literature to link AKI to long-term mortality after MI.[29] The trial by Fox et al. revealed a striking association between in-hospital bleeding events and worsening AKI despite lower rates of usage of oral and intravenous antiplatelet agents.[26] There are several implications of the findings of the trial by Fox et al.:

- Treating physicians must be made aware of the fact that prevalence of AKI is high in patients with AMI
- Increase in in-hospital mortality and bleeding is observed even with marginal rise in serum creatinine

- Impact of AKI in AMI can be gauged by the fact that despite absence of risk factors like shock, cardiac surgery, and pre-existing CKD, in-hospital mortality increases due to AKI alone
- Acute kidney injury as a marker of risk in AMI is independent of the fact of whether CAG is done or nephrotoxic contrast is used.

STEMI, ACS AND CKD

Many large registries report that almost 40% of the patients with NSTEMI and 30% of the patients with STEMI have CKD as defined by eGFR of <60 mL/min/1.73 m^2.[30] CKD portends a worsened prognosis in patients with CAD. Accelerated atherogenesis and underlying uremic state along with traditional and nontraditional risk factors are responsible for this worse prognosis.[30] Same worse prognosis is also demonstrated in the setting of ACS and kidney disease. In fact, presence of kidney disease doubles the mortality in patients with ACS. This mortality rate is second only to cardiogenic shock and congestive heart failure.[31] They used the US Renal Data System database and examined 34,189 patients on long-term dialysis after a first episode of AMI. This study demonstrated in-hospital mortality of 26% and 1-year and 2-year mortality rate of 59% and 73%, respectively. Mueller et al.[32] in their study consisting of 1,400 consecutive patients analyzed correlation between baseline renal function and long-term mortality after NSTEMI-ACS. In this study, patients with an eGFR of <60 mL/min/1.73 m^2 had a higher in-hospital as well as long-term mortality. This study confirmed that baseline renal function is a strong independent predictor of in-hospital and long-term mortality, irrespective of the method used for revascularization. This finding applies to patients with NSTEMI-ACS treated early with PCI. The absence of overall benefit in this subset of patients is probably explained by PCI-related complications that may overweigh advantages created by revascularization like CIN, coronary stent thrombosis, and restenosis.

However, since patients with CKD are not included in most of the randomized control trials, evidence-based data with established or newer drugs and interventional strategies are lacking in this subgroup of populations.

PROGNOSTIC RELEVANCE OF CKD IN ACS

Even though it is known that CKD represents a potent and independent risk factor for poor outcome in ACS, the underlying mechanism for the worse prognosis is far from clear. However, following factors may be operating:
- Interplay between extensive comorbidities
- More severe disease on presentation with ACS
- Suboptimal utilization of available and known cardioprotective therapies.
- Less aggressive treatment
- Frequent errors in dosing lead to excess toxicity from conventional therapies
- Unique pathobiology of CKD.

Recently, important differences between extent of coronary atherosclerosis and coronary plaque morphology in patients with and without CKD have been demonstrated.[33] Coronary lesions in CKD patients were longer with greater luminal encroachment and with a higher plaque burden than in non-CKD counterparts. Some studies using radiofrequency intravascular ultrasound (IVUS) have demonstrated that renal dysfunction not only results in greater plaque burden and luminal encroachment but also modulates the plaque composition to less stable phenotype. It has also been demonstrated that CKD plays an important role in left ventricular remodeling after MI through enhanced inflammatory response and oxidative stress.[34]

■ TREATMENT OF PATIENTS WITH ACS AND CKD

Treatment of ACS in patients with CKD is particularly problematic and poses unique challenges. To date, scarce data is available for treating ACS in patients with CKD. This is primarily because, traditionally, patients with CKD on dialysis were not included in any randomizing controlled trials evaluating interventional and standard medical therapy for ACS. So far, no optimal treatment strategy is defined for this subgroup of patients.

■ CORONARY REPERFUSION STRATEGIES

There is no clarity yet on how the patients with CKD should be treated during early phase of STEMI. The primary concerns are regarding how aggressively the reperfusion should be attempted by employing standard techniques such as PCI or intravenous thrombolytic agents. Even though many landmark trials such as GUSTO trial and the International Study of Infarct Survival have amply demonstrated the effectiveness of thrombolytic agents in reducing mortality due to STEMI, no subgroup analysis was performed in patients with CKD.[35]

In a study by Wright et al.[36] 13% of the total population received intravenous fibrinolytic therapy and 10% received PCI as primary treatment. Reperfusion therapy was used less frequently in patients with CKD— indicating a treatment bias in favor of patients with less advanced renal dysfunction. In a study by Beattie et al. use of thrombolytic agents and PCI decreased with progressive decline in renal function.[37] The potential development of CIN and higher mortality may be a rational explanation of lesser use of PCI in this group of patients. However, the potential risk of bleeding episodes is just a partial justification for decreased use of thrombolytic agents in CKD patients.

Chronic kidney disease should not preclude the success rate of PCI or pharmacological reperfusion even though there is an increased risk of major adverse events. A single-center retrospective study was conducted to evaluate the effects of an invasive management in patients with STEMI and kidney disease (serum creatinine ranging from 1.2 to 2.8 mg/dL).[38] All of these patients received thrombolytic therapy, while early PCI or coronary bypass surgery was performed in 47% and 28% of patients with normal renal function and 32% and 30% of those with CKD. In this study, patients with CKD showed a higher mortality when compared to patients with normal renal function. However, 30-day and 6-month mortality was reduced from 22% to 4% among CKD patients who underwent PCI during hospitalization. This study confirms that even though mild-to-moderate CKD in the setting of STEMI is associated with increased mortality, early PCI may be beneficial in this group of patients.

Worse outcomes have been reported in patients with CKD who are treated with PCI by Late Angioplasty Complications Trial and others.[39,40] As a result, the best strategy for STEMI patients with CKD remains elusive in spite of clear reported benefits from pharmacological and mechanical coronary reperfusion in the setting of STEMI. Recently, regardless of the treatment with primary PCI (29%), thrombolysis (32%), or medical therapy (31.5), GRACE registry has shown similar in-hospital mortality rates in STEMI patients with advanced CKD.[41]

In a broad conclusion, it may be said that primary PCI may be beneficial with mild-to-moderate renal dysfunction but does not confer benefit in severe CKD.

Invasive treatment is considered superior to an initial conservative treatment in the setting of NSTEMI-ACS. Similarly, early invasive treatment is thought to be better than a delayed invasive treatment. Decreased mortality was reported in the KAMIR study when an invasive strategy was adopted within 24 hours after admission as opposed to conservative strategy, except in those with severe CKD.[42] The same KAMIR study reported that early invasive strategy yielded better results when compared to delayed invasive treatment in patients with CKD. However, this tendency decreased as renal function decreased.[42]

■ STANDARD MEDICAL THERAPY

Many studies have confirmed that patients with ACS are treated less aggressively when they have a concomitant CKD. These studies also reveal that aggressiveness of treatment of ACS parallels the degree of impairment of renal function and many proven beneficial therapies are underutilized, despite increased prevalence of hypertension, CCF, and CAD and despite the proven benefits of survival in the patients with normal renal function. Berger et al.[43] confirmed in their study of 1,025 patients with STEMI and on chronic dialysis that β-blockers, aspirin and ACE inhibitors were less likely to be used in patients on dialysis in spite of the fact these patients are considered as "ideal candidates" for the use of these medications. However, the authors of this study found similar benefits of these drugs in patients on dialysis and also in those who were not on dialysis.

Berger et al. when comparing the dialysis and nondialysis groups, observed an absolute reduction in short-term mortality with aspirin, β-blocker and ACE-inhibitor therapy. As much as 21% absolute reduction in mortality was associated with aspirin use in dialysis groups.[43] The same figure stood at 23% in nondialysis groups. When β-blocker therapy was used, 14% absolute reduction in mortality was reported in dialysis as well as nondialysis groups. The ACE inhibitor use was associated with a 16% absolute reduction in 30-day mortality in patients subjected to dialysis and a 5% reduction in nondialysis patients.

■ ANTITHROMBOTIC THERAPY

Judicious use of antithrombotic agents among CKD patients in a setting of ACS is a daunting challenge and the refinement of such therapy is far from achieved. On one hand, normal aggregation and adherence of platelets are affected in CKD patients. On the other hand, a hypercoagulation state is noticed in patients with CKD with high level of Von Willebrand factors fibrinogen and thrombin generation. A combination of these factors puts these patients at risk for vascular thrombosis and hemorrhage at the same time. Therefore, well-established antiplatelet drugs such as aspirin and clopidogrel should be weighed against risk of bleeding in patients with renal dysfunction. Since maximum benefits of the antiplatelet agents are observed in the setting of NSTEMI-ACS setting, it is advisable to keep the CKD patients on aspirin therapy with a suggestion for low dose. A recent meta-analysis found that low-dose aspirin (65–260 mg/day) was found to be as efficacious as high-dose aspirin therapy (325 mg) for secondary prevention of CAD in patients of with CKD and ESRD.[2,29] The currently prevailing practice guidelines suggest adding to aspirin another antiplatelet agent such as ticlopidine, clopidogrel, prasugrel, or ticagrelor for treatment of high-risk patients of ACS. Clinical evidence was provided that ticagrelor is a more effective antiplatelet agent than clopidogrel in patients with ACS in the Platelet Inhibition and Patient Outcomes Study. Efficacy of ticagrelor over clopidogrel was proved regardless of renal function and without any need for reduction of dose to prevent major bleeding.[44]

However, a recent meta-analysis found that in the patients of CKD, benefits of antiplatelet therapy are outweighed by risks of major bleeding.[45] In addition to antiplatelet agents, heparin is in wide use in patients with ACS. There are two preparations of heparin available—the unfractionated heparin (UFH) and low-molecular weight heparin (LMWH). However, optimal dosing of enoxaparin, a type of LMWH, is not yet established in CKD patients. A retrospective study showed significant incidence of bleeding and even death among the CKD patients treated with enoxaparin.[46] It suggests that fine adjustment of dosage is needed in these patients to minimize the risk of bleeding. Until conclusive results are available regarding optimal dosing, it may be safer to use UFH in CKD patients presenting with ACS.

Use of antiplatelet agents such as platelet GP IIb/IIIa receptor inhibitors has become the mainstay of anticoagulation for high-risk patients of NSTEMI-ACS undergoing PCI. However, since the patients with CKD were not included in most randomized controlled trials investigating GP IIb/IIIa antagonists, it is not clear whether CKD patients will derive similar benefit and safety advantage from these drugs when compared to patients with normal renal function. Since abciximab is excreted by renal system, its use in CKD is recommended while tirofiban and eptifibatide, excreted by kidneys, need to be avoided.[47]

■ STATINS IN ACS PATIENTS WITH CKD

Data collected from a trial on 300,823 patients of the National Registry of Myocardial Infarction suggest that administration of statins within 24 hours after hospitalization for AMI lowers the rate of early complications and in-hospital mortality. This beneficial effect is probably due to the pleiotropic effects of statins.[48] Stains are known to dampen inflammation, ED and coagulation disorders observed after MI.[48] Despite ample evidence, statins are less likely to be used for ACS in patients with CKD. The reason for this reluctance to use statins is not clear. Concerns for further renal damage and other toxic side effects may be the probable explanation. In addition, since the patients with CKD are likely to harbor other comorbidities, contraindications for the use of statins may increase. Another probable reason for the reduced use of statins is that come uncertainty lingers regarding their therapeutic benefits in patients with kidney disease. No clear evidence is found in patients of CKD regarding a positive relationship between blood cholesterol and cardiovascular events. Since chronic malnutrition and inflammation are common in severe CKD, the blood cholesterol levels ultimately drop in CKD patients. This "U"-shaped relationship between dyslipidemia and cardiovascular events in patients with CKD and CHD is often described as "low-cholesterol paradox".[49] This paradox has raised suspicion regarding utility of lipid-lowering therapy. In addition, some concerns about drug toxicity due to high-dose statins persist in patients of CKD. Increased risk of myopathy is reported due to use of statin in patients with kidney dysfunction.

However, a recent study of Heart and Renal Protection Trial has shown that combination of ezetimibe and low-dose statins can safely reduce the risk of major atherosclerotic events in a wide range of patients with CKD—including patients on dialysis.[17]

PHARMACOLOGICAL TREATMENT OF STABLE ANGINA IN PATIENTS ON DIALYSIS

- As in patients without CKD, the choice of antianginal agent depends on presence or absence of comorbidities. Specific issues to the patients on dialysis include appropriate dosage
- Hemoglobin levels should be targeted in the range of 10–11 g/dL for the patients who are on erythropoiesis-stimulating agents for correction of anemia
- Aspirin should be administered in a low dose of 81 mg/day. Patients on dialysis who choose to avoid risk of bleeding may forego aspirin all together.

PHARMACOLOGICAL TREATMENT OF UNSTABLE ANGINA IN PATIENTS ON DIALYSIS

- Most of the drugs used to treat unstable angina and ACS can be used in patients with or without renal failure. If there are no contraindications, aspirin, β-blockers, ACE inhibitors, ARBs (angiotensin II receptor blockers), and nitroglycerin, statins should be given in appropriate dose
- Platelet GP IIb/IIIa inhibitors should be administered whenever indicated and if there are no contraindications after taking into account the possibility of bleeding episodes. Abciximab is the preferred agent in patients with renal failure because it does not require dosage adjustment. Marked dosage adjustment of tirofiban is required in patients on dialysis, while eptifibatide is contraindicated
- In order to reduce the risk of hypotension and arrhythmias, the timing and performance of HD session in the setting of ACS should focus on maintaining hemodynamic stability, lowering of bleeding risk, and minimizing fluctuations of electrolytes
- If indicated and in the absence of any contraindications, fibrinolytic and antithrombolytic agents, heparin and/or platelet GP IIa/IIIb inhibitors should be administered to patients on dialysis
- Invasive strategies such as PCI or coronary artery bypass graft (CABG) can be performed in dialysis patients as in general population.

STEMI in Renal Transplant

Gupta et al. in their retrospective study over 10-year period from 2003 to 2013 observed that renal transplant recipients were less likely to receive reperfusion compared with patients without CKD, but had similar risk-adjusted in-hospital mortality but more long-term mortality.[50] In contrast, compared with patients with stage 5D CKD, renal transplant recipients were much more likely to receive reperfusion and had markedly lower in-hospital mortality rates. They suggested the approach in treatment in the renal transplant patients should be similar to that general population.

CARDIAC BIOMARKERS IN CKD: POINTS OF RELEVANCE[51]

- Whenever a patient presents with clinical, EKG, or imaging findings suspicious of MI, cardiac troponins I and T (cTnI and cTnT) are the preferred biomarkers for the diagnosis of myocardial injury in patients with CKD
- Troponins are preferred to MB (muscle/brain) isoenzymes of creatine kinase (CK-MB) because of their superior specificity and sensitivity
- Rather than a single value at the time presentation, a serial change (either a rise or a fall) in troponin concentrations should be used to diagnose AMI
- It is not clear whether troponin-based criteria for diagnosis of AMI in patients with CKD should be any different in patients without CKD. Among patients in whom all troponin levels are at or above the 99th percentile, a greater than 20% change in serially measured troponin is an acceptable threshold range for a positive diagnosis of AMI in patients with CKD. However, there is no data to support this approach to diagnose AMI
- CK-MB should not be used to diagnose AMI when cardiac troponin is available because CK-MB is less sensitive and specific for myocardial injury
- Increased level of troponin is an independent prognosticator after AMI in patients with CKD as in general population
- Increased levels of troponin in stable and asymptomatic patients of CKD suggest worse long-term cardiovascular outcomes and poor survival.

CONTRAST-INDUCED NEPHROPATHY

- An absolute (>0.5 mg/dL) or relative (>25%) increase in serum creatinine with respect to baseline within 48–72 hours of contrast injection is defined as CIN. However, the increase in serum levels of creatinine must be in the absence of alternative causes for it to be defined as CIN
- Since CIN is generally short-lasting and histopathologic changes caused by underlying renal dysfunction complicate biopsy assessment, the pathophysiology of CIN is not well understood. Renal vasoconstriction and acute tubular injury are some of the important mechanisms
- CIN is the third most common reason for hospital-acquired AKI. It is related to short- as well as long-term mortality and morbidity
- *Risk factors*: Chronic kidney disease with serum creatinine of >1.5 mg/dL or eGFR of <60 mL/min/1.73 m^2 is the most important risk factor for CIN. Diabetes mellitus, hypovolemia, hypotension, advanced age heart failure, anemia, nephrotoxic drug use, hyperuricemia, and high-quantity or recent (within 10 days) use of contrast media are some of the other risk factors
- The greater the number of risk factors a person has, the greater their risk for CIN

- A registry[52] has shown that PCI is likely to yield better outcomes when compared to no PCI at all in the setting of obstructive CAD with unstable angina, STEMI, heart failure, and who have a concomitant CKD. Therefore, certain procedures such as PCI should not be avoided whenever necessary, even if there is a risk of CIN. However, a second procedure such as percutaneous angioplasty should be avoided, if possible, within 10 days of a first procedure such as a diagnostic coronary angiogram. If such a step is not practical in a particular institute, at least 3 days must be allowed to lapse between the two procedures
- Maximum of 30 mL contrast for diagnostic coronary angiogram and 100 mL for PCI may be used[53]
- Procedures involving intra-arterial contrast are prone for CIN when compared to intravenous contrast medium[54]
- Patients with near-normal renal function are at low risk for CIN. A few precautions are warranted in such a setting apart from avoidance or correction of volume depletion.

Following preventive measures are suggested to avoid CIN:
- Use iodixanol or low-osmolar agents such as iopamidol or ioversol instead of iohexol. High-osmolar agents (1,400–1,800 mOsmol/kg) should be avoided
- Use lower dose of contrast and avoid repetitive and closely spaced tests (e.g. <48 h apart)
- Avoid volume depletion and nonsteroidal anti-inflammatory drugs (NSAIDs). If renal dysfunction sets in (serum creatinine: ≥1.5 mg/dL or eGFR: ≤60 mL/min/1.73 m^2), it is prudent to discontinue metformin 2 days prior to contrast injection and remain off metformin for 2 days after the procedure.[55]

It is recommended to use intravenous fluids, preferably isotonic saline, prior to and continued after intravenous injection of contrast in patients with high risk for CIN—defined as eGFR of <45 mL/min/1.73 m^2, proteinuria, diabetes, and other comorbidities. Patients should be given sodium bicarbonate 1 hour before the procedure as 3 mL/kg/h or isotonic sodium chloride 6–12 hours prior to the procedure. Adequate hydration must continue with 1 mL/kg/h for 6–12 hours after the procedure. The hydration must be extended for some more period in hot weather or in advanced cases of CKD.
- All patients at risk may not be given acetylcysteine. 1,200 mg of NAC (N-acetylcysteine) through oral route 1 day before the procedure and a day after is the well-accepted protocol. NAC should be given twice daily from then on
- There is no role for prophylactic HD. Hemofiltration is suggested in patients with stage-5 kidney disease.

Epilogue

- Acute and CKD are bad prognostic markers in CAD in general and ACS in particular
- Risk factor management in CAD patients with CKD is on similar lines as the general population
- Medical management of patients with CKD and ACS also is similar to non-CKD patients with a few exceptions:
  - Aspirin to be used in low dose of 81 mg
  - Ticagrelor is preferred over clopidogrel
  - Unfractionated heparin is preferred over enoxaparin
  - Abciximab is preferred over tirofiban and eptifibatide to be avoided
- Fear of CIN should not deter the treating cardiologist from doing PCI in ACS and heart failure
- STEMI and NSTEMI patients with mild-to-moderate CKD should be given benefit of early PCI but those with severe CKD may be managed conservatively
- Appropriate measures to prevent CIN in high-risk individuals should be undertaken
- ACS in renal transplant recipients may be treated like that in general population.

REFERENCES

1. Anavekar NS, McMurray JJ, Velazquez EJ, et al. Relation between renal dysfunction and cardiovascular outcomes after myocardial infarction. N Engl J Med. 2004;351(13): 1285-95.
2. Tonelli M, Wiebe N, Culleton B, et al. Chronic kidney disease and mortality risk: a systematic review. J Am Soc Nephrol. 2006;17(7):2034-47.
3. Stenvinkel P, Carrero JJ, Axelsson J, et al. Emerging biomarkers for evaluating cardiovascular risk in the chronic kidney disease patient: how do new pieces fit into the uremic puzzle? Clin J Am Soc Nephrol. 2008;3(2):505-21.
4. Charytan DM, Stern NM, Mauri L. CKD and coronary collateral supply in individuals undergoing coronary angiography after myocardial infarction. Clin J Am Soc Nephrol. 2012;7(7):1079-86.
5. Shioi A, Taniwaki H, Jono S, et al. Mönckeberg's medial sclerosis and inorganic phosphate in uremia. Am J Kidney Dis. 2001;38(4 Suppl 1):S47-9.
6. Stenvinkel P, Chung SH, Heimbürger O, et al. Malnutrition, inflammation, and atherosclerosis in peritoneal dialysis patients. Perit Dial Int. 2001;21(Suppl 3):S157-62.
7. Caliskan Y, Demirturk M, Ozkok A, et al. Coronary artery calcification and coronary flow velocity in haemodialysis patients. Nephrol Dial Transplant. 2010;25(8):2685-90.
8. Park MJ, Jung JI, Oh YS, et al. Assessment of epicardial fat volume with threshold-based 3-dimensional segmentation in CT: comparison with the 2-dimensional short axis-based method. Korean Circ J. 2010;40(7):328-33.
9. Chronic Kidney Disease Prognosis Consortium, Matsushita K, van der Velde M, et al. Association of estimated glomerular filtration rate and albuminuria with all-cause and cardiovascular mortality in general population cohorts: a collaborative meta-analysis. Lancet. 2010;375(9731):2073-81.
10. Matsushita K, Coresh J, Sang Y, et al. Estimated glomerular filtration rate and albuminuria for prediction of cardiovascular outcomes: a collaborative meta-analysis of individual participant data. Lancet Diabetes Endocrinol. 2015;3(7):514.

11. van der Velde M, Matsushita K, Coresh J, et al. Lower estimated glomerular filtration rate and higher albuminuria are associated with all-cause and cardiovascular mortality. A collaborative meta-analysis of high-risk population cohorts. Kidney Int. 2011;79(12):1341-52.
12. Sarnak MJ, Levey AS, Schoolwerth AC, et al. Kidney disease as a risk factor for development of cardiovascular disease: a statement from the American Heart Association Councils on Kidney in Cardiovascular Disease, High Blood Pressure Research, Clinical Cardiology, and Epidemiology and Prevention. Circulation. 2003;108(17):2154-69.
13. Tonelli M, Muntner P, Lloyd A, et al. Risk of coronary events in people with chronic kidney disease compared with those with diabetes: a population-level cohort study. Lancet. 2012;380(9844):807-14.
14. Wattanakit K, Coresh J, Muntner P, et al. Cardiovascular risk among adults with chronic kidney disease, with or without prior myocardial infarction. J Am Coll Cardiol. 2006;48(6):1183-9.
15. Foley RN, Wang C, Collins AJ. Cardiovascular risk factor profiles and kidney function stage in the US general population: the NHANES III study. Mayo Clin Proc. 2005;80(10):1270-7.
16. Kaysen GA, Eiserich JP. The role of oxidative stress-altered lipoprotein structure and function and microinflammation on cardiovascular risk in patients with minor renal dysfunction. J Am Soc Nephrol. 2004;15(3):538-48.
17. Baigent C, Landray MJ, Reith C, et al. The effects of lowering LDL cholesterol with simvastatin plus ezetimibe in patients with chronic kidney disease (Study of Heart and Renal Protection): a randomised placebo-controlled trial. Lancet. 2011;377(9784):2181-92.
18. Mann JF, Gerstein HC, Pogue J, et al. Renal insufficiency as a predictor of cardiovascular outcomes and the impact of ramipril: the HOPE randomized trial. Ann Intern Med. 2001;134(8):629-36.
19. Blood Pressure Lowering Treatment Trialists' Collaboration, Ninomiya T, Perkovic V, et al. Blood pressure lowering and major cardiovascular events in people with and without chronic kidney disease: meta-analysis of randomised controlled trials. BMJ. 2013;347:f5680.
20. Fox CS, Muntner P, Chen AY, et al. Use of evidence-based therapies in short-term outcomes of ST-segment elevation myocardial infarction and non-ST-segment elevation myocardial infarction in patients with chronic kidney disease: a report from the National Cardiovascular Data Acute Coronary Treatment and Intervention Outcomes Network registry. Circulation. 2010;121(3):357-65.
21. Palmer SC, Di Micco L, Razavian M, et al. Antiplatelet agents for chronic kidney disease. Cochrane Database Syst Rev. 2013;(2):CD008834.
22. Washam JB, Herzog CA, Beitelshees AL, et al. Pharmacotherapy in chronic kidney disease patients presenting with acute coronary syndrome: a scientific statement from the American Heart Association. Circulation. 2015;131(12):1123-49.
23. Freeman RV, Mehta RH, Al Badr W, et al. Influence of concurrent renal dysfunction on outcomes of patients with acute coronary syndromes and implications of the use of glycoprotein IIb/IIIa inhibitors. J Am Coll Cardiol. 2003;41(5):718-24.
24. Newsome BB, Warnock DG, McClellan WM, et al. Long-term risk of mortality and end-stage renal disease among the elderly after small increases in serum creatinine level during hospitalization for acute myocardial infarction. Arch Intern Med. 2008;168(6):609-16.
25. Karkouti K, Wijeysundera DN, Yau TM, et al. Acute kidney injury after cardiac surgery: focus on modifiable risk factors. Circulation. 2009;119(4):495-502.
26. Fox CX, Muntner P, Chen AY, et al. Short-term Outcomes of Acute Myocardial Infarction in Patients with Acute Kidney Injury: A Report from the National Cardiovascular Data Registry. Circulation. 2012;125(3):497-504.

27. Goldberg A, Hammerman H, Petcherski S, et al. In-hospital and 1-year mortality of patients who develop worsening renal function following acute ST-elevation myocardial infarction. Am Heart J. 2005;150(2):330-7.
28. Weisbord SD, Chen H, Stone RA, et al. Associations of increases in serum creatinine with mortality and length of hospital stay after coronary angiography. J Am Soc Nephrol. 2006;17(10):2871-7.
29. Parikh CR, Coca SG, Wang Y, et al. Long-term prognosis of acute kidney injury after acute myocardial infarction. Arch Intern Med. 2008;168(9):987-95.
30. Sarnak MJ, Levey AS, Schoolwerth AC, et al. Kidney disease as a risk factor for development of cardiovascular disease: a statement from the American Heart Association Councils on Kidney in Cardiovascular Disease, High Blood Pressure Research, Clinical Cardiology, and Epidemiology and Prevention. Hypertension. 2003;42(5):1050-65.
31. Masoudi FA, Plomondon ME, Magid DJ, et al. Renal insufficiency and mortality from acute coronary syndromes. Am Heart J. 2004;147(4):623-9.
32. Mueller C, Neumann FJ, Perruchoud AP, et al. Renal function and long-term mortality after unstable angina/non-ST segment elevation myocardial infarction treated very early and predominantly with percutaneous coronary intervention. Heart. 2004;90(8):902-7.
33. Baber U, Stone GW, Weisz G, et al. Coronary plaque composition, morphology, and outcomes in patients with and without chronic kidney disease presenting with acute coronary syndromes. JACC Cardiovasc Imaging. 2012;5(3 Suppl):S53-61.
34. Naito K, Anzai T, Yoshikawa T, et al. Impact of chronic kidney disease on postinfarction inflammation, oxidative stress, and left ventricular remodeling. J Card Fail. 2008; 14(10):831-8.
35. James SK, Lindahl B, Siegbahn A, et al. N-terminal pro-brain natriuretic peptide and other risk markers for the separate prediction of mortality and subsequent myocardial infarction in patients with unstable coronary artery disease: a Global Utilization of Strategies to Open occluded arteries (GUSTO)-IV substudy. Circulation. 2003;108(3):275-81.
36. Wright RS, Reeder GS, Herzog CA, et al. Acute myocardial infarction and renal dysfunction: a high-risk combination. Ann Intern Med. 2002;137(7):563-70.
37. Beattie JN, Soman SS, Sandberg KR, et al. Determinants of mortality after myocardial infarction in patients with advanced renal dysfunction. Am J Kidney Dis. 2001;37(6): 1191-200.
38. Hobbach HP, Gibson CM, Giugliano RP, et al. The prognostic value of serum creatinine on admission in fibrinolytic-eligible patients with acute myocardial infarction. J Thromb Thrombolysis. 2003;16(3):167-74.
39. Tonbul HZ, Demir M, Altintepe L, et al. Malnutrition-inflammation-atherosclerosis (MIA) syndrome components in hemodialysis and peritoneal dialysis patients. Ren Fail. 2006;28(4):287-94.
40. Corradi D, Maestri R, Callegari S, et al. The ventricular epicardial fat is related to the myocardial mass in normal, ischemic and hypertrophic hearts. Cardiovasc Pathol. 2004;13(6):313-6.
41. Medi C, Montalescot G, Budaj A, et al. Reperfusion in patients with renal dysfunction after presentation with ST-segment elevation or left bundle branch block: GRACE (Global Registry of Acute Coronary Events). JACC Cardiovasc Interv. 2009;2(1):26-33.
42. Hachinohe D, Jeong MH, Saito S, et al. Management of non-ST-segment elevation acute myocardial infarction in patients with chronic kidney disease (from the Korea Acute Myocardial Infarction Registry). Am J Cardiol. 2011;108(2):206-13.
43. Berger AK, Duval S, Krumholz HM. Aspirin, beta-blocker, and angiotensin-converting enzyme inhibitor therapy in patients with end-stage renal disease and an acute myocardial infarction. J Am Coll Cardiol. 2003;42(2):201-8.

44. James S, Budaj A, Aylward P, et al. Ticagrelor versus clopidogrel in acute coronary syndromes in relation to renal function: results from the Platelet Inhibition and Patient Outcomes (PLATO) trial. Circulation. 2010;122(11):1056-67.
45. Palmer SC, Di Micco L, Razavian M, et al. Effects of antiplatelet therapy on mortality and cardiovascular and bleeding outcomes in persons with chronic kidney disease: a systematic review and meta-analysis. Ann Intern Med. 2012;156(6):445-59.
46. Fernandez JS, Sadaniantz BT, Sadaniantz A. Review of antithrombotic agents used for acute coronary syndromes in renal patients. Am J Kidney Dis. 2003;42(3):446-55.
47. Freeman RV, Mehta RH, Al Badr W, et al. Influence of concurrent renal dysfunction on outcomes of patients with acute coronary syndromes and implications of the use of glycoprotein IIb/IIIa inhibitors. J Am Coll Cardiol. 2003;41(5):718-24.
48. Fonarow GC, Wright RS, Spencer FA, et al. Effect of statin use within the first 24 hours of admission for acute myocardial infarction on early morbidity and mortality. Am J Cardiol. 2005;96(5):611-6.
49. Foley RN, Parfrey PS, Sarnak MJ. Epidemiology of cardiovascular disease in chronic renal disease. J Am Soc Nephrol. 1998;9:S16-S23.
50. Gupta T, Kolte D, Khera S, et al. Management and Outcomes of ST-Segment Elevation Myocardial Infarction in US Renal Transplant Recipients. JAMA Cardiol. 2017;2(3):250-8.
51. deFilippi C, Henrich WL. (2018). Serum cardiac biomarkers in patients with renal failure. [online] Available from https://www.uptodate.com/contents/serum-cardiac-biomarkers-in-patients-with-renal-failure. [Last accessed May, 2019].
52. Reddan DN, Klassen PS. Chronic kidney disease and cardiovascular risk: Time to focus on therapy. J Am Soc Nephrol. 2002;13(9):2415-6.
53. Mehran R, Aymong ED, Nikolsky E, et al. A simple risk score for prediction of contrast-induced nephropathy after percutaneous coronary intervention: development and initial validation. J Am Coll Cardiol. 2004;44(7):1393-9.
54. Rudnick MR. (2018). Prevention of contrast nephropathy associated with angiography. [online] Available from https://www.uptodate.com/contents/prevention-of-contrast-nephropathy-associated-with-angiography. [Last accessed May, 2019].
55. Thomsen HS. European Society of Urogenital Radiology (ESUR) guidelines on the safe use of iodinated contrast media. Eur J Radiol. 2006;60(3):307-13.

CHAPTER 4

Acute Coronary Syndrome Patients needing Anticoagulation

Prologue
Two Plus Two may not be Four

A 72-year-old gentleman presented with anterior wall ST segment elevation myocardial infarction (STEMI). He was on dabigatran for atrial fibrillation (AF) with international normalized ratio (INR) of 1.6.

A 58-year-old patient who had undergone aortic valve replacement presented with acute anterior wall STEMI and heart failure. His INR was 1.9.

Main cause of worry was bleeding during primary percutaneous coronary intervention (PCI) or subsequently as triple antithrombotic therapy though ideal to prevent ischemic events but may do so at the cost of increased bleeding.

The issues before me were:
- Go ahead with primary PCI or treat conservatively
- Radial or femoral access?
- If primary PCI what should be periprocedural anticoagulation?
  - None
  - Heparin
  - Bivalirudin.
- Bare-metal stent (BMS) or drug-eluting stent (DES)
- Long-term antithrombotic regimen
  - Dual antiplatelet therapy (DAPT)
  - DAPT with vitamin K antagonists (VKAs)
  - DAPT with direct oral thrombin antagonists (DOTAs).

The author did primary PCI in both the patients with 5,000 units of IV heparin. Both patients subsequently were put on triple antithrombotic therapy.

The overall prevalence of AF is steadily increasing in the general population. Significant amount of cardiovascular mortality and morbidity is attributed to AF leading to stroke and thromboembolism.[1,2] Keeping this in mind, many of the guidelines recommend oral anticoagulants (OACs) as prophylaxis in almost all the patients with AF with a moderate to high risk of developing stroke.[3-5] As much as 5–15% of the patients with AF are known to undergo PCI sometime in their life span.[3]

Similarly, about 5–15% of the patients undergoing PCI are to known to harbor AF.[6] DAPT are invariably given to prevent stent thrombosis in almost all patients undergoing PCI and stent implantation. Therefore, a combination of antithrombotic therapy including OAC agents and antiplatelet agents is given to the patients with AF and who are subjected to PCI and stent implantation. However, some concerns are usually expressed regarding the clinical benefit of intensive combination antithrombotic therapy because of the propensity for fatal hemorrhage. The fatal bleeding event may offset the benefit of reducing the risk of ischemic damage.[7]

Park et al. in their study observed an increasing trend of AF patients undergoing PCI[1] (Flowchart 1 and Fig. 1). They also observed a rising and changing trend of anticoagulation treatment over 10 years.[1]

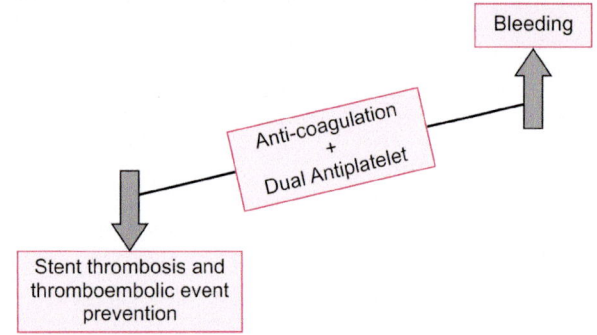

FLOWCHART 1: A balancing act.

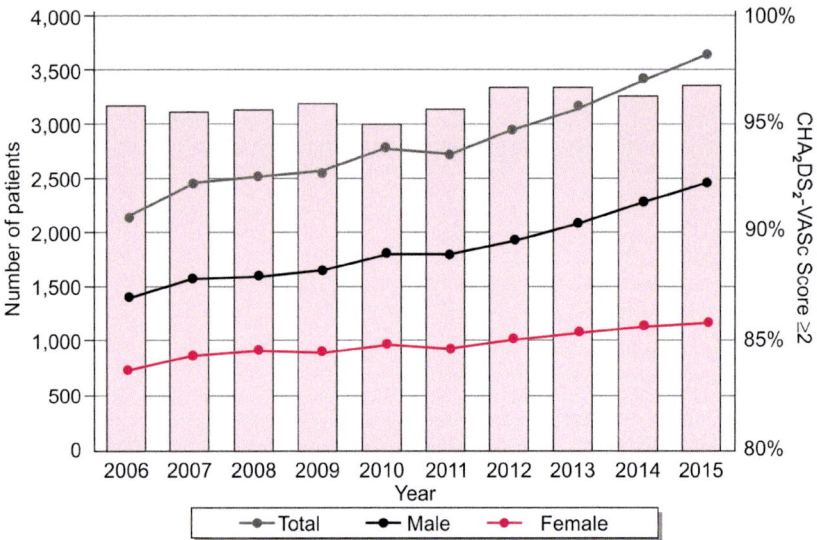

FIG. 1: The number of AF patients undergoing PCI over 10 years (p <0.001).

Source: Park J, Choi EK, Han KD, et al. Temporal trends in prevalence and antithrombotic treatment among Asians with atrial fibrillation undergoing percutaneous coronary intervention: a nationwide Korean population-based study. PLoS One. 2019;14(1):e0209593.

PRIMARY PCI VERSUS CONSERVATIVE TREATMENT

The study by Alonso et al. in subanalysis of the Global Registry of Acute Coronary Events (GRACE) describes the clinical and treatment characteristics of patients on chronic OAC presenting with STEMI.[8] They observed that the patients on OAC appeared to be less likely to undergo Cath/PCI, to receive antiplatelet and antithrombotic medications, or to receive other evidence-based therapies compared with STEMI patients not on chronic OAC. The patients on OAC carried a higher risk of adverse cardiac events. This coupled with the fact that they were less likely to receive ideal reperfusion therapy [primary PCI, coronary artery bypass grafting (CABG)] or therapy in the recommended time frame put them at additional disadvantage.

They compared users of OACs who underwent PCI to nonusers of OAC. They observed that major hemorrhagic event occurred more frequently in OAC users who underwent cath-angio or PCI. On the contrary, such hemorrhagic episodes were less frequent in the patients on conservative line and with medications. However, hospital mortality rate was higher among the patients treated conservatively (Fig. 2). As much as 20% of the medically treated patients succumbed within 6 months. This mortality

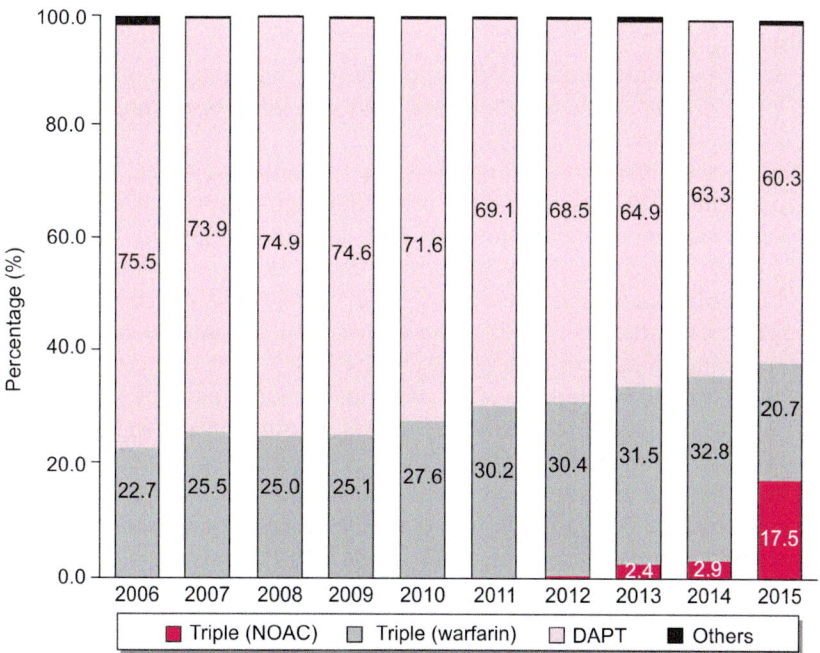

FIG. 2: The trend of anticoagulation treatment over 10 years.

Source: Park J, Choi EK, Han KD, et al. Temporal trends in prevalence and antithrombotic treatment among Asians with atrial fibrillation undergoing percutaneous coronary intervention: a nationwide Korean population-based study. PLoS One. 2019;14(1):e0209593.

figure was just 6.9% in those patients who were subjected to PCI. Similarly, 6-month mortality was also lower when primary PCI was done. This was true irrespective of the time frame in which PCI was done.

Thus, primary PCI should be offered to patients of STEMI on OAC.

■ RADIAL VERSUS FEMORAL ACCESS

There is some persistent controversy regarding the preferred approach to arterial access while performing primary PCI for acute coronary syndrome (ACS). Both of these approaches were noted to be equally safe and efficacious in RIVAL study.[9] However, the radial approach was associated with some mortality benefit in a subgroup analysis of STEMI patients.[9] MATRIX trial in ACS patients too showed less major bleeding and mortality in radial versus femoral route.[10] Moreover, radial access was associated with reduced bleeding and vascular complications in many studies on patients with uninterrupted warfarin therapy undergoing PCI and who had a mean INR of 2.4.[11]

■ PERIPROCEDURAL ANTICOAGULATION

The most effective regimen of anticoagulation during periprocedural period for patients with ACS is not yet defined. Any such regimen must prevent ischemic complications without augmenting the risk for major bleeding episode:

- The therapeutic range of INR for patients on warfarin is 2.0–3.0. PCI is apparently safe in these patients and there is usually no need for additional periprocedural anticoagulation[12]
- At present, there are no large studies proving the safety and efficacy of performing PCI on non-VKA oral anticoagulants (NOACs) without additional anticoagulation. Until such a time, it is recommended to give additional heparin or bivalirudin and avoid glycoprotein (GP) IIb/IIIa inhibitors irrespective of the dose of NOAC. This is particularly true for those patients of STEMI where thrombogenic state is exaggerated compared to patients undergoing elective PCI[13]
- The risk of major bleeding when additional anticoagulants or antiplatelet agents are given to patients of STEMI is theoretically higher when the patients have taken a NOAC within 4 hours of presentation when compared to those who have taken the same NOAC >12 hours prior to presentation. Whenever heparin is used as the additional anticoagulant, target activated clotting time (ACT) levels (250–300 s) can be used for the purpose of titrating heparin dose. This can be done even in those patients who are on regular NOAC[13]
- *Heparin versus bivalirudin*: When compared to heparin alone or heparin combined with GP IIb/IIIa inhibitors, bivalirudin is noted to have significantly reduced risk of major bleeding as revealed in multiple trials.[14] Hence, it may be prudent to use bivalirudin instead of heparin in patients

who have taken their last dose of NOAC within 4 hours of presentation. It is also recommended in elderly patients with impaired renal function
- *Acute antiplatelet treatment*: Compared to clopidogrel, the likelihood of major bleeding is significantly higher when ticagrelor or prasugrel is used.[15] Therefore, a loading dose of clopidogrel (600 mg) is preferable to the newer antiplatelet agents.

LONG-TERM ANTIPLATELET AND ANTICOAGULATION TREATMENT

Trials
- Dual and triple therapy with warfarin: WOEST[16]
- Dual and triple therapy with direct oral anticoagulants (DOACs): PIONEER AF-PCI,[17] RE-DUAL PCI.[18]

WOEST Trial
This is an open-label, randomized, controlled trial comparing use of clopidogrel with or without aspirin in patients taking OAC therapy and subjected to PCI. The authors of this trial concluded that compared to triple therapy with warfarin:
- Dual therapy with clopidogrel and OAC causes less bleeding
- Dual therapy with clopidogrel and OAC did not increase thrombotic events.

In their meta-analysis of DOAC trials (PIONEER AF-PCI, RE-DUAL PCI), Brunetti et al. observed that first, the use of DOACs is generally safer than and as effective as warfarin in such patients; second, dual therapy with DOACs is as safer than and as effective as triple therapy with warfarin; third, dual therapy with DOACs is as safe as and as effective as triple therapy with DOACs in patients with AF treated with PCI.[19]

Before embarking on long-term antiplatelet/anticoagulant treatment after PCI individual patient's thrombotic and bleeding risks need to be assessed.

Thrombotic Risk
Risk factors for a thrombotic (or ischemic) event (e.g. myocardial infarction, stroke that is often secondary to AF, need for repeat revascularization, or cardiovascular death) after PCI include recent ACS or stroke; complicated, multivessel coronary artery disease (CAD), particularly in patients with diabetes, a suboptimal result at the time of PCI, the need to prematurely stop antithrombotic therapy, age ≥65 years, prior stent thrombosis, and chronic kidney disease.

Bleeding Risk (Box 1)[20]
The following are recommendations for antiplatelet/anticoagulation treatment during the first 6–12 months after PCI in patients needing anticoagulation other than those with mechanical valves (Flowcharts 2 and 3):

BOX 1: Score to calculate bleeding risk.[20]

- For >160 mm Hg systolic (uncontrolled hypertension) score obtained is +1
- For >2 X normal with AST/ALP/AP >3 X (abnormal liver function, cirrhosis or bilirubin) normal score obtained is +1
- For >2.26 mg/dL or 200 μmol/L (abnormal renal function dialysis, transplant, Cr) score obtained is +1
- For stroke score obtained is +1
- For bleeding (prior major bleeding or predisposition to bleeding) score obtained is +1
- For labile INR (unstable/high INR) time in therapeutic range <60% score obtained is +1
- For elderly >65 score obtained is +1
- For drugs like concomitant, antiplatelet, aspirin, clopidogrel, NSAIDs score obtained is +1
- For drugs like concomitant excess alcohol use ≥8 drink/week score obtained is +1

0–2 Low bleed risk
3–4 High bleed risk
\> Very high bleed risk

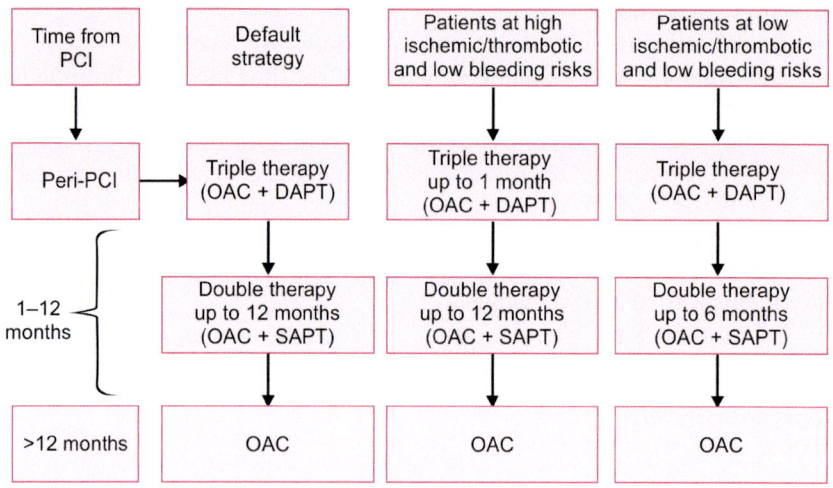

(DAPT: dual antiplatelet therapy; OAC: oral anticoagulant; PCI: percutaneous coronary intervention; SAPT: single antiplatelet therapy)

FLOWCHART 2: 2018 AHA North American consensus white paper.

- For patients at low thrombotic and low bleeding risk, DOAC (dabigatran 150 mg twice) with *clopidogrel* plus *aspirin* (triple therapy) alternatively DOAC plus clopidogrel (dual therapy) may be chosen. If triple therapy is chosen, it is continued for 1-6 months and then aspirin is dropped. Clopidogrel 75 mg daily is continued for 6-12 months

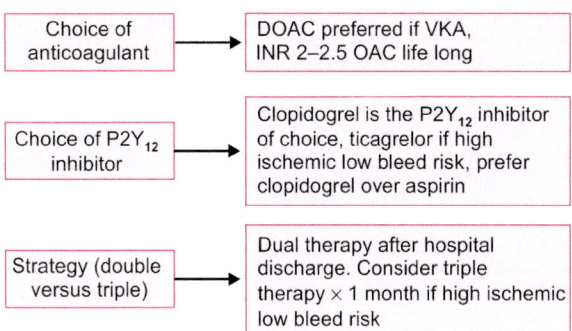

(DOAC: direct oral anticoagulant; INR: international normalized ratio; OAC: oral anticoagulant; VKA: vitamin K antagonist)

FLOWCHART 3: 2018 Expert Consensus.

- For patients at low thrombotic and high bleeding risk, initial treatment with DOAC (dabigatran 110 mg twice a day) plus *clopidogrel* 75 mg daily is preferred regimen for 6-12 months
- For patients at high thrombotic and low bleeding risk, the author and his colleagues suggest initial treatment with DOAC (dabigatran 150 mg twice a day) plus *clopidogrel* plus *aspirin* (triple therapy) is suggested for 1-6 months after which aspirin is discontinued and DOAC and clopidogrel continued till 12 months after PCI
- For patients at high thrombotic and bleeding risk, individualized patient decision making is essential.

After 12 months only OACs may be continued unless there is high thrombotic risk when single antiplatelet therapy (SAPT) is added.

Patients with heart valves

In patients with mechanical heart valves, non-VKA oral anticoagulants (DOACs) should not be considered alternatives to therapy with VKA and should not be used. They are contraindicated.

■ BARE-METAL STENT OR DRUG-ELUTING STENTS?

The ZEUS trial[21] which compared Zotarolimus DES and BMS and SENIOR trial[22] which compared any new DES with BMS and DAPT given for 1 month in both groups observed that new current generation DES are superior to BMS.

Epilogue
- Patients on anticoagulants who present with STEMI benefit from primary PCI albeit at the cost of increased bleeding
- Radial access is preferred especially if INR is more than 2.5 mainly to reduce major bleeding events

- When patient is on VKA if INR is therapeutic (between 2 and 3), periprocedure anticoagulation may not be needed
- When patient is on DOAC, it is safer to anticoagulate notwithstanding the fact if the last dose of DOAC is within 4 hours risk of bleeding is higher
- Bivalirudin may be preferred to heparin especially in patients with increased risk of bleeding
- Current generation DES is preferred over BMS
- Vitamin K antagonists have no substitute when patient has mechanical valve
- Long-term antithrombotic treatment is determined by individual's thrombotic/bleeding risk
  - High thrombotic risk demands triple antithrombotic therapy and even up to 6 months and in low thrombotic risk patients SAPT with anticoagulation might suffice
  - In high bleeding risk patients, clopidogrel with anticoagulation may be used
- In triple antithrombotic therapy, DOAC especially dabigatran is preferred over VKA unless patient is well maintained on VKA for long time
- In triple antithrombotic or SAPT with anticoagulant therapy, clopidogrel/ticagrelor is preferred over aspirin.

REFERENCES

1. Park J, Choi EK, Han KD, et al. Temporal trends in prevalence and antithrombotic treatment among Asians with atrial fibrillation undergoing percutaneous coronary intervention: a nationwide Korean population-based study. PLoS One. 2019;14(1):e0209593.
2. Lee SR, Choi EK, Han KD, et al. Trends in the incidence and prevalence of atrial fibrillation and estimated thromboembolic risk using the CHA2DS2-VASc score in the entire Korean population. Int J Cardiol. 2017;236:226-31.
3. Kirchhof P, Benussi S, Kotecha D, et al. 2016 ESC guidelines for the management of atrial fibrillation developed in collaboration with EACTS. Eur J Cardiothorac Surg. 2016;50(5):e1-88.
4. January CT, Wann LS, Alpert JS, et al. 2014 AHA/ACC/HRS guideline for the management of patients with atrial fibrillation: executive summary: a report of the American College of Cardiology/American Heart Association Task Force on practice guidelines and the Heart Rhythm Society. Circulation. 2014;130(23):2071-104.
5. Valgimigli M, Bueno H, Byrne RA, et al. 2017 ESC focused update on dual antiplatelet therapy in coronary artery disease developed in collaboration with EACTS: the Task Force for dual antiplatelet therapy in coronary artery disease of the European Society of Cardiology (ESC) and of the European Association for Cardio-Thoracic Surgery (EACTS). Eur Heart J. 2018;39(3):213-60
6. Choi HI, Ahn JM, Kang SH, et al. Prevalence, management, and long-term (6-year) outcomes of atrial fibrillation among patients receiving drug-eluting coronary stents. JACC Cardiovasc Interv. 2017;10(11):1075-85.
7. Dans AL, Connolly SJ, Wallentin L, et al. Concomitant use of antiplatelet therapy with dabigatran or warfarin in the Randomized Evaluation of Long-Term Anticoagulation Therapy (RE-LY) trial. Circulation. 2013;127(5):634-40.
8. Alonso A, Gore JM, Awad HH, et al. Management and outcomes of patients presenting with STEMI by use of chronic oral anticoagulation: results from the GRACE registry. Eur Heart J Acute Cardiovasc Care. 2013;2(3):280-91.

9. Jolly SS, Yusuf S, Cairns J, et al. Radial versus femoral access for coronary angiography and intervention in patients with acute coronary syndromes (RIVAL): a randomised, parallel group, multicentre trial. Lancet. 2011;377:1409-20.
10. Valgimigli M, Gagnor A, Calabró P, et al. Radial versus femoral access in patients with acute coronary syndromes undergoing invasive management: a randomised multicentre trial. Lancet. 2015;385:2465-76.
11. Baker NC, O'Connell EW, Htun WW, et al. Safety of coronary angiography and percutaneous coronary intervention via the radial versus femoral route in patients on uninterrupted oral anticoagulation with warfarin. Am Heart J. 2014;168:537-44.
12. Karjalainen PP, Vikman S, Niemelä M, et al. Safety of percutaneous coronary intervention during uninterrupted oral anticoagulant treatment. Eur Heart J. 2008;29:1001-10.
13. Heidbuchel H, Verhamme P, Alings M, et al. Updated European Heart Rhythm Association Practical Guide on the use of non-vitamin K antagonist anticoagulants in patients with non-valvular atrial fibrillation. Europace. 2015;17(10):1467-507.
14. Valgimigli M, Frigoli E, Leonardi S, et al. Bivalirudin or unfractionated heparin in acute coronary syndromes. N Engl J Med. 2015;373:997-1009.
15. Wallentin L, Becker RC, Budaj A, et al. Ticagrelor versus clopidogrel in patients with acute coronary syndromes. N Engl J Med. 2009;361:1045-57.
16. Dewilde WJ, Oirbans T, Verheugt FW, et al. Use of clopidogrel with or without aspirin in patients taking oral anticoagulant therapy and undergoing percutaneous coronary intervention: an open-label, randomised, controlled trial. Lancet. 2013;381:1107-15.
17. Gibson CM, Mehran R, Bode C, et al. Prevention of bleeding in patients with atrial fibrillation undergoing PCI. N Engl J Med. 2016;375:2423-34.
18. Cannon CP, Bhatt DL, Oldgren J, et al. Dual antithrombotic therapy with dabigatran after PCI in atrial fibrillation. N Engl J Med. 2017;377:1513-24.
19. Brunetti ND, Tarantino N, De Gennaro L, et al. Direct oral anticoagulants versus standard triple therapy in atrial fibrillation and PCI: meta-analysis. Open Heart. 2018;5:e000785.
20. Pisters R, Lane DA, Nieuwlaat R, et al. A novel user-friendly score (HAS-BLED) to assess 1-year risk of major bleeding in patients with atrial fibrillation. Chest. 2010;138(5):1093-100.
21. Valgimigli M, Patialiakas A, Thury A, et al. Zotarolimus-eluting versus bare-metal stents in uncertain drug-eluting stent candidates. J Am Coll Cardiol. 2015;65:805-15.
22. Varenne O, Cook S, Sideris G, et al. Drug-eluting stents in elderly patients with coronary artery disease (SENIOR): a randomised single-blind trial. Lancet. 2018;391:41-50.

CHAPTER 5

Acute Coronary Syndrome with Chronic Obstructive Pulmonary Disease

Prologue

Huffing and Puffing: Lung or Heart?

On a cold December evening last year, a frail-looking, 40-year-old man, walked into my consulting room—flanked and supported by a middle-aged lady with wrinkles of worry writ large on her face. He coughed incessantly and he was a little short of breath. He was being treated by a general physician for chronic obstructive pulmonary disease (COPD) for long time and now he was referred to me for recent worsening of dyspnea. The author did not find anything amiss on echocardiography but the patient was markedly dyspneic on treadmill right in the stage I. Even though the telltale signs of myocardial ischemia were not detected on his electrocardiogram, the author decided to conduct a coronary angiogram (CAG) the following day. The CAG revealed a tight stenosis of left anterior descending artery (LAD)—occluding almost 90% of its lumen.

However, the author was in a quandary now. Should the author subject the patient to angioplasty? Is his dyspnea due to respiratory disease (COPD) or cardiac disease (LAD stenosis)? What if he is not relieved of dyspnea even after the revascularization procedure? These were some of the questions that troubled me. However, after explaining every eventuality in detail to his relatives and obtaining their written consent, the author decided to proceed with angioplasty. To everyone's pleasant surprise, his dyspnea reduced remarkably during the first few days after the procedure. Almost 2 years down the line, although he has symptoms of COPD and he is not breathless on his daily activities. In hindsight, although this patient had COPD and his recent worsening was due to ischemia. This experience prompted me to read more and sift through the available literature on cardiac disease associated with comorbid conditions such as COPD.

■ INTRODUCTION

Chronic obstructive pulmonary disease is widely prevalent across the population. The unstressed fact is that cardiovascular disease is the most common mode of death in COPD patients. As evident from many trials,

COPD has been found to be an independent risk factor for cardiovascular mortality.[1] In fact it may contribute to major, i.e. between 22% and 39% of the deaths.[1,2] This was the observation of many large trials like Lung Health Study, Towards a Revolution in COPD Health, Understanding Potential Long-term Impacts on Function with Tiotropium, European Respiratory Society Study on Chronic Obstructive Pulmonary Disease and Inhaled Steroids in Obstructive Lung Disease in Europe (ISOLDE).[1,2] Yet these patients receive suboptimal care for acute myocardial infarction (AMI) both in hospital and later as is revealed in many studies and in an elegant review by KJ Rothnie.[3] Patients with COPD not only have increased mortality and rehospitalization rates after AMI but also tend to have poor health status. Recent studies have thrown some light into possible mechanisms contributing to the excessive cardiovascular risk conferred in COPD patients. These could be oxidative stress, endothelial dysfunction, arterial stiffness, increased inflammation and thrombotic predisposition.[1]

▪ CHRONIC OBSTRUCTIVE PULMONARY DISEASE AND CORONARY ARTERY DISEASE

Several studies have suggested that the most common though less recognized cause of death in COPD patients is coronary artery disease (CAD). In fact, the Tucson epidemiologic study of airway obstructive disease has found that cardiovascular disease is responsible for half of deaths in patients of COPD, being true even in patients with severe airway obstruction.[4,5]

The natural history of COPD involves episodes of acute exacerbations. These episodes of acute exacerbations in COPD constitute an important causative factor for not only mortality during hospitalization for acute event long-term mortality as well. This is mainly because of associated cardiovascular disease which has significant impact in pathogenesis as well prognosis of COPD exacerbations. This theory finds support in the study of Donaldson et al.[6] who have shown that during acute exacerbations of COPD risk of acute cardiovascular events increase. Several retrospective studies have demonstrated increase in troponin levels during acute exacerbations of COPD.[7,8] There is a suggestion that they might reflect severity of exacerbation rather than occurrence of true myocardial infarction (MI) and may even be a marker for increased postdischarge mortality.[7,8] These facts drive home a message that the treatment of acute exacerbation of COPD not only entails respiratory but should also be directed toward early recognition of acute ischemic event for its prompt treatment.

▪ PRESENTING FEATURES IN ACUTE MYOCARDIAL INFARCTION

Patients who present in the hospital with AMI have the prevalence of chronic pulmonary disease (COPD) to the tune of 10–17%.[9-12]

This is definitely underestimated because of presence of undiagnosed COPD. When pulmonary function tests are done in hospitalized patients, the prevalence goes up as shown by Nemick et al.[13] As reported in various studies, COPD patients who have MI have atypical symptoms like breathlessness, atypical chest pain, and palpitations rather than typical retrosternal pain.[9-11] Therefore as reported in MINAP study [Myocardial Ischaemia National Audit Project, a national register for all MI and acute coronary syndrome (ACS) admissions in the United Kingdom] as high as 25–50% patients will have diagnosis other than MI or ACS in patients who later had the diagnosis as MI.[1] This study further observed that MI patients with COPD and higher in-hospital and 6-month mortality. These findings held true even after adjustment for associated comorbidities, demographics or other medication use. Delay in the diagnosis of MI in COPD patients led to delay in starting reperfusion therapies like primary percutaneous coronary intervention (PCI) or thrombolysis. Similarly COPD patients are more likely to present with non-ST segment elevation myocardial infarction (NSTEMI) than ST segment elevation myocardial infarction (STEMI). They also have lower cardiac biomarker levels of troponins and creatine kinase-MB (CK-MB) levels.[12,14-16] In one study, COPD has been associated with late presentation >12 hours after onset of symptoms.[16]

■ DIAGNOSIS AND MANAGEMENT OF ACUTE MYOCARDIAL INFARCTION

Atypical presenting symptoms of AMI lead to either delayed diagnosis or the diagnosis may be totally missed. Amongst the patients who get admitted in the hospital with acute exacerbation of COPD around 8% patients meet the criteria for the diagnosis of MI as mentioned in the universal definition of MI.[17] It is still not very clear whether this is misdiagnosis or it is true MI triggered because of COPD exacerbation. Similarly in patients admitted for COPD around 33% are found to have had prior episode of MI which has not been documented before and thus patient is unaware of its occurrence.[18] This is especially more prevalent in female population.[18] As revealed from the data from the MINAP, a national register for all MI and ACS admissions in the United Kingdom, Rothnie et al. have provided interesting insights into fact of increased mortality following first MI in patients of COPD.[12] The delayed diagnosis of STEMI in patients with COPD led to delayed definitive reperfusion therapy. This is mainly responsible for increased mortality of STEMI in COPD patients, as when adjustments were made for this diagnostic and therapeutic delay and in-hospital mortality was roughly cut in half and no longer statistically significant in whom primary PCI was done. This register goes on to show that COPD patients have reduced usage of standard secondary preventive measures after STEMI like the use of β-blockers. This is the main cause of increased 6-month mortality in patients of COPD who develop MI. This, now, is nearly established fact that in patients of COPD who develop MI, β-blockers started either before or after STEMI is associated with improved survival.[19] Adoption of proven secondary preventive measures like β-blockers and angiotensin-converting enzyme (ACE) inhibitors has shown to markedly decrease 6-month mortality (from 43% down to 25%) in patients of STEMI with COPD. As with STEMI, patients of COPD who develop NSTEMI also have atypical presentation leading to delayed diagnosis, delayed definitive treatment like PCI and hence higher in-hospital and 6-month mortality. As in patients of STEMI when adjustments were made for the diagnostic and therapeutic delay, adoption of secondary preventive measures has markedly attenuated in-hospital and 6-month mortality (roughly by 50%) however, unlike STEMI patients in NSTEMI with COPD patients the mortality difference continues to be statistically significant for both in hospital and 6 months mortality.[1]

■ CHRONIC OBSTRUCTIVE PULMONARY DISEASE AND CORONARY REVASCULARIZATION

ST Segment Elevation Myocardial Infarction

Like MINAP, other studies from the United Kingdom and Sweden too have observed that COPD patients developing STEMI are less likely to be treated with definitive reperfusion strategies like primary PCI.[3,10] This was further corroborated by earlier US studies.[11,16]

However, there is definite change in thinking, change in practice over the time leading to increasing use of primary PCI in patients of COPD developing STEMI. This is the observation of recent US study which did not find any difference in the use of primary PCI in patients with or without COPD.[15]

Non-ST Segment Elevation Myocardial Infarction

As previously mentioned, patients of COPD have atypical presentation leading to delayed diagnosis of NSTEMI. Furthermore, these patients are less likely to receive angiography despite carrying increased risk as underscored by different studies.[10-12,15,16] This observation persisted even when adjustments were made for age, frailty, coexistence of other comorbid conditions.[12]

The NSTEMI guidelines recommend angiography within 72 hours for those with more than or equal to 3% risk of death at 6 months as per the risk evaluation scores.[20,21] Early percutaneous intervention has been shown to significantly improve outcome in high-risk patients, those with the highest risk being the most to gain.[22,23]

Coronary Artery Bypass Grafting versus Coronary Angioplasty

Besides medical treatment, myocardial revascularization in the form of coronary artery bypass grafting (CABG) or PCI has been the mainstay of the treatment in patients with CAD. While CABG surgery has been established as the form of treatment since 1960s, after its advent recently PCI now is the preferred revascularization procedure because of its minimally invasive nature.[24] Both procedures carry major technical differences. CABG surgery has the advantage of providing complete revascularization even in vessels relatively small for stenting, in complex, calcified, chronically occluded vessels not suitable for angioplasty. A well-performed CABG with arterial revascularization has shown to have lasting results with long-term vessel patency. In select group of patients like left main and three-vessel disease with left ventricular dysfunction, CABG has also been shown to improve survival. The down side of CABG surgery is thoracotomy/sternotomy and sometimes extracorporeal circulation which may be a concern in COPD patients. As against CABG, PCI is less invasive with fewer acute complications, short hospital stay. Main concern with PCI is restenosis in first 6–8 months. This has been reduced to nearly 5–7% with latest generation drug-eluting stents but not eliminated completely. PCI has been definitely shown to reduce symptoms, improve quality of life but with regards to its effect on reduction of MI or improvement of survival there is no solid evidence.

Like any pulmonary morbidity, COPD carries an independent risk for CABG surgery which involves sternotomy or thoracotomy and sometimes extracorporeal circulation. COPD is also a risk factor for long-term cardiovascular events in CAD patients undergoing revascularization. This makes COPD an inherent part of any score which predicts risk.

Nishiyama et al. studied and analyzed consecutive patients who underwent either CABG or PCI in patients who had COPD.[25] They found COPD patients carried high cardiac and all-cause mortality in both group of patients. Selvaraj et al. studied patients of COPD who underwent only PCI in both elective and in primary setting.[26,27] Their observation was similar in that COPD patients carry higher risk than those without COPD.

Thus, it can be concluded that COPD patients carry high risk and have suboptimal results after undergoing revascularization be CABG or PCI.

■ LONG-TERM TREATMENT IN COPD PATIENTS WITH MYOCARDIAL INFARCTION

As previously mentioned, patients with COPD who have MI are treated suboptimally. They are also likely to have higher comorbidity profile. Based on multiple randomized trials, various current guidelines have recommended different drug therapies for secondary prevention after an episode of AMI. These include β-blocker, an ACE inhibitor or angiotensin receptor blocker, a statin, and dual antiplatelet therapy (aspirin indefinitely and P2Y12 receptor antagonist for 1 year).[20,21]

Beta-blockers

There is a general belief that in COPD patients β-blockers are contraindicated for the fear of causing or aggravating bronchospasm resulting from smooth muscle contraction caused by unopposed action of alpha-1 receptors. Repeated studies have failed to show change in forced expiratory volume in 1 second (FEV1), or exacerbating COPD.[28] This is explained on the basis of cardioselective β-blockers are acting selectively at cardiac β1 receptors with no action on bronchial β2 receptors, precluding the unopposed activation of alpha-1 adrenergic receptors. As shown in meta-analysis of β-blockers in COPD, it is clear that they have mortality benefit.[29]

Despite this information, there is still hesitation on the part of physicians to prescribe β-blockers as secondary prevention after AMI.[10-12,16]

The under use of recommended secondary preventive drugs is also applicable to other medicines like ACE inhibitor or angiotensin receptor blocker, statins (only exception being P2Y12 receptor antagonists) which are less often prescribed in MI patients with COPD than those without COPD.[10-12,14-16] However, here the difference is not as glaring as with β-blockers.

Angiotensin-converting Enzyme Inhibitor in COPD

The concern with the use of ACE inhibitors in patients with COPD was whether they will aggravate cough and whether they will have same secondary prevention benefit as those without COPD.

Mortensen et al. studied the effect of prior usage of ACE inhibitors in patients of COPD admitted with acute exacerbation. They found that prior ACE inhibitor use was associated with decreased mortality at 90 days.[30] Similarly Kathleen Packard has attempted to assess the incidence of cough and bronchial responsiveness in patients of congestive heart failure, COPD or asthma. She has reviewed available literature in this regard. Her conclusion was ACE inhibitors do not increase the incidence of cough or bronchoconstriction in patients with primary airway disease like COPD or asthma.[22]

Statins in Chronic Obstructive Pulmonary Disease

Mortensen et al. studied the effect of prior statin usage in patients of COPD admitted for acute exacerbation. They found that in COPD patients prior statin use in patients hospitalized for acute exacerbation was associated with decreased mortality at 90 days.[30]

Chao Cao et al. have extensively reviewed the literature in their meta-analysis studying the effect of statins on COPD exacerbations, cardiovascular events and COPD mortality. After this thorough review in their meta-analysis, they concluded that statin usage reduced incidence of MI, reduced cardiovascular mortality, reduced COPD mortality and also all-cause mortality. Their another surprise conclusion was reduction in the incidence of COPD exacerbations and as a consequence hospitalization.[23]

Antiplatelets and Chronic Obstructive Pulmonary Disease

Chronic obstructive pulmonary disease as seen previously is a chronic inflammatory state. As a result, there is increased platelet activity raising a speculation that this might increase thrombotic cardiovascular events. This may provide a role for antiplatelet therapy to reduce the ischemic events and hence the mortality. There are some studies in this regard.

Pavasini et al. performed a systematic review and meta-analysis including patients with COPD and found that all-cause mortality was significantly lower with antiplatelet treatment.[31]

Ivabradine

Ivabradine is a latest addition to the armamentarium. This compound selectively inhibits if current of sinoatrial node myocytes thereby selectively reducing heart rate without any other effect on cardiovascular system unlike β-blockers. Heart rate is one of the major determinants of myocardial oxygen consumption. Therefore, ivabradine by reducing heart rate has the potential of reducing ischemic burden. Ivabradine does not have other autonomic effects of β-blockers which too reduce heart rate. These include fatigue, vasoconstriction, changes in blood pressure, sexual dysfunction, etc. These side effects of β-blockers may be of particular concern in fragile COPD patients. In fact, some studies have shown that ivabradine has favorable ischemia related outcomes and in addition prevents adverse vascular remodeling in CAD.[32]

It is encouraging fact that over the time this treatment difference in patients of AMI with or without COPD is narrowing as the awareness is growing. As mentioned above in the United States of America, now COPD patients with STEMI are treated with primary PCI and usage of β-blockers as secondary prevention has also increased.[15] This is in contrast to Europe wherein COPD patients with STEMI still do not receive these recommended treatment.[10-12,15]

■ POSSIBLE MECHANISMS LINKING CORONARY ARTERY DISEASE AND CHRONIC OBSTRUCTIVE PULMONARY DISEASE

Both CAD and COPD have some risk factors in common like smoking. However, increased prevalence of CAD in patients of COPD appears independent of the common risk factors.[33] COPD itself being a chronic inflammatory state has been shown by different studies as a risk factor for atherosclerosis and development for CAD.[34] It has been suggested that the risk conferred by COPD for CAD may surpass the risk because of conventional risk factors like hypertension and hypercholesterolemia.[34]

Still the exact mechanism linking CAD with COPD is elusive, but systemic inflammation, oxidative stress and hypoxemia may be the most likely candidates.[35-40]

> ## Epilogue
> - Prevalence of COPD is increasing
> - Chronic obstructive pulmonary disease is an independent marker of morbidity and mortality in patients with CAD
> - Coronary artery disease is widely prevalent in patients with COPD and is the major cause of mortality and yet is underdiagnosed
> - Acute coronary syndrome has atypical presentation in patients with COPD, hence the diagnosis is missed or delayed
> - Acute coronary syndrome in COPD carries higher morbidity and mortality because of delayed diagnosis and under treatment
> - Chronic obstructive pulmonary disease influences morbidity in patients undergoing CABG surgery
> - Percutaneous coronary intervention including primary PCI has been shown to be beneficial even in patients with COPD
> - All the secondary prevention strategies in CAD hold true even in COPD patients
> - Beta-blockers (withheld due to concern of bronchospasm) and ACE inhibitors (withheld due to concern of cough) should be prescribed whenever indicated in patients with CAD.

REFERENCES

1. Rajagopalan S, Brook RD. Mortality from myocardial infarction in chronic obstructive pulmonary disease: minding and mending the 'Gap'. Heart. 2015;101(14):1085-6.
2. Berry CE, Wise RA. Mortality in COPD: causes, risk factors, and prevention. COPD. 2010;7:375-82.
3. Rothnie KJ, Quint JK. Chronic obstructive pulmonary disease and acute myocardial infarction: effects on presentation, management and outcomes. Eur Heart J Qual Care Clin Outcomes. 2016;2(2):81-90.
4. Camilli AE, Robbins DR, Lebowitz MD. Death certificate reporting of confirmed airways obstructive disease. Am J Epidemiol. 1991;133:795-800.
5. Hansell AL, Walk JA, Soriano JB. What do chronic obstructive pulmonary disease patients die from? A multiple cause coding analysis. Eur Respir J. 2003;22:809-14.
6. Donaldson GC, Hurst JR, Smith CJ, et al. Increased risk of myocardial infarction and stroke following exacerbation of COPD. Chest. 2010;137:1091-7.
7. Harvey MG, Hancox RJ. Elevation of cardiac troponins in exacerbation of chronic obstructive pulmonary disease. Emerg Med Australas. 2004;16:212-5.
8. Brekke PH, Omland T, Holmedal SH, et al. Troponin T elevation and long-term mortality after chronic obstructive pulmonary disease exacerbation. Eur Respir J. 2008;31:563-70.
9. Hadi HA, Zubaid M, Al Mahmeed W, et al. Prevalence and prognosis of chronic obstructive pulmonary disease among 8,167 Middle Eastern patients with acute coronary syndrome. Clin Cardiol. 2010;33:228-35.
10. Andell P, Koul S, Martinsson A, et al. Impact of chronic obstructive pulmonary disease on morbidity and mortality after myocardial infarction. Open Heart. 2014;1:e000002.

11. Stefan MS, Bannuru RR, Lessard D, et al. The impact of COPD on management and outcomes of patients hospitalized with acute myocardial infarction: a 10-year retrospective observational study. Chest. 2012;141:1441-8.
12. Rothnie KJ, Smeeth L, Herrett E, et al. Closing the mortality gap after a myocardial infarction in people with and without chronic obstructive pulmonary disease. Heart. 2015;101:1103-10.
13. Nemick DB, Matyushin GV, Protopopov AV, et al. Results of treatment of acute ST-segment elevation myocardial infarction in patients with chronic obstructive pulmonary disease: data of a retrospective, single-center study (in-hospital period). Rational Pharmacother Card. 2015;11(6):561-70.
14. Salisbury AC, Reid KJ, Spertus JA. Impact of chronic obstructive pulmonary disease on post-myocardial infarction outcomes. Am J Cardiol. 2007;99:636-41.
15. Enriquez JR, de Lemos JA, Parikh SV, et al. Association of chronic lung disease with treatments and outcomes patients with acute myocardial infarction. Am Heart J. 2013;165:43-9.
16. Bursi F, Vassallo R, Weston SA, et al. Chronic obstructive pulmonary disease after myocardial infarction in the community. Am Heart J. 2010;160:95-101.
17. McAllister DA, Maclay JD, Mills NL, et al. Diagnosis of myocardial infarction following hospitalisation for exacerbation of COPD. Eur Respir J. 2012;39:1097-103.
18. Brekke PH, Omland T, Smith P, et al. Underdiagnosis of myocardial infarction in COPD—Cardiac Infarction Injury Score (CIIS) in patients hospitalised for COPD exacerbation. Respir Med. 2008;102:1243-7.
19. Quint JK, Herrett E, Bhaskaran K, et al. Effect of β blockers on mortality after myocardial infarction in adults with COPD: population based cohort study of UK electronic healthcare records. BMJ. 2013;347:f6650.
20. Hamm CW, Bassand JP, Agewall S, et al. ESC guidelines for the management of acute coronary syndromes in patients presenting without persistent ST-segment elevation: the Task Force for the management of acute coronary syndromes (ACS) in patients presenting without persistent ST-segment elevation of the European Society of Cardiology (ESC). Eur Heart J. 2011;32:2999-3054.
21. National Institute for Health and Clinical Excellence. Unstable angina and NSTEMI: the early management of unstable angina and non-ST-segment-elevation myocardial infarction. London: Royal College of Physicians (UK); 2010.
22. Packard KA, Wurdeman RL, Arouni AJ. ACE inhibitor-induced bronchial reactivity in patients with respiratory dysfunction. Ann Pharmacother. 2002;36:1058-67.
23. Cao C, Wu Y, Xu Z, et al. The effect of statins on chronic obstructive pulmonary disease exacerbation and mortality: a systematic review and meta-analysis of observational research. Sci Rep. 2015;5:16461.
24. Wijns W, Kolh P, Danchin N, et al. Guidelines on myocardial revascularization: the Task Force on Myocardial Revascularization of the European Society of Cardiology (ESC) and the European Association for Cardio-Thoracic Surgery (EACTS). Eur Heart J. 2010;31:2501-55.
25. Nishiyama K, Morimoto T, Furukawa Y, et al. Chronic obstructive pulmonary disease—an independent risk factor for long-term cardiac and cardiovascular mortality in patients with ischemic heart disease. Int J Cardiol. 2010;143:178-83.
26. Selvaraj CL, Gurm HS, Gupta R, et al. Chronic obstructive pulmonary disease as a predictor of mortality in patients undergoing percutaneous coronary intervention. Am J Cardiol. 2005;96:756-9.
27. Campo G, Saia F, Guastaroba P, et al. Prognostic impact of hospital readmissions after primary percutaneous coronary intervention. Arch Intern Med. 2011;171:1948-9.
28. Salpeter SR, Ormiston TM, Salpeter EE, et al. Cardioselective beta-blockers for chronic obstructive pulmonary disease: a meta-analysis. Respir Med. 2003;97:1094-101.

29. Etminan M, Jafari S, Carleton B, et al. Beta-blocker use and COPD mortality: a systematic review and meta-analysis. BMC Pulm Med. 2012;12:48.
30. Mortensen EM, Copeland LA, Pugh MJ, et al. Impact of statins and ACE inhibitors on mortality after COPD exacerbations. Respir Res. 2009;10:45.
31. Pavasini R, Biscaglia S, d'Ascenzo F, et al. Antiplatelet treatment reduces all-cause mortality in COPD patients: a systematic review and meta-analysis. COPD. 2016;13(4):509-14.
32. Boschetto P, Beghé B, Fabbri LM, et al. Link between chronic obstructive pulmonary disease and coronary artery disease: implication for clinical practice. Respirology. 2012;17(3):422-31.
33. Mannino DM, Thorn D, Swensen A, et al. Prevalence and outcomes of diabetes, hypertension and cardiovascular disease in COPD. Eur Respir J. 2008;32:962-9.
34. Hole DJ, Watt GC, Davey-Smith G, et al. Impaired lung function and mortality risk in men and women: findings from the Renfrew and Paisley prospective population study. BMJ. 1996;313:711-5; discussion 715-6.
35. Sin DD, Man SF. Why are patients with chronic obstructive pulmonary disease at increased risk of cardiovascular diseases? The potential role of systemic inflammation in chronic obstructive pulmonary disease. Circulation. 2003;107:1514-9.
36. Barnes PJ, Celli BR. Systemic manifestations and comorbidities of COPD. Eur Respir J. 2009;33:1165-85.
37. Hurst JR, Wilkinson TM, Perera WR, et al. Relationships among bacteria, upper airway, lower airway, and systemic inflammation in COPD. Chest. 2005;127:1219-26.
38. De Martinis M, Franceschi C, Monti D, et al. Inflamm-ageing and lifelong antigenic load as major determinants of ageing rate and longevity. FEBS Lett. 2005;579:2035-9.
39. De Martinis M, Franceschi C, Monti D, et al. Inflammation markers predicting frailty and mortality in the elderly. Exp Mol Pathol. 2006;80:219-27.
40. Barnes PJ. Chronic obstructive pulmonary disease: effects beyond the lungs. PLoS Med. 2010;7:e1000220.

CHAPTER 6

Acute Coronary Syndrome with Chronic Liver Disease

■ TO STENT OR NOT TO STENT IS THE QUESTION!

Prologue

A few months back, an elderly gentleman in his late sixties with multiple ailments was admitted in the hospital where the author work. He was popular and well known to the inner circle of our hospital management. He suffered from advanced liver cirrhosis along with multiple complications of long-standing diabetes mellitus. He had a large amount of free fluid in the peritoneal cavity—indicating obvious liver failure. He had nephropathy, retinopathy and recurrent variceal bleed requiring multiple attempts at ligation. In addition, his platelet count was 30,000/mL which was dangerously low. Even though he did not display any obvious signs of myocardial ischemia, the electrocardiogram showed multiple arrhythmias. A subsequent coronary angiogram (CAG) revealed a hemodynamically significant stenosis in the right coronary artery (RCA)—requiring angioplasty. However, this situation posed a treatment dilemma. Following were the issue before me:

- Can the author prescribe dual platelet agents after the stenting in this patient with a low platelet count of 30,000/mL and past history of variceal bleeding?
- Since this patient was being considered for liver transplantation which necessitates discontinuation of all antiplatelet agents, should the author go ahead with stenting—even risking the possibility of in-stent thrombosis in the immediate future?
- If at all the author decide to stent the stenotic lesion, what type of stent the author should be using—bare-metal stent or the drug-eluting stent?

Just a few days later, another patient with advanced liver cirrhosis presented to me with cardiac arrest due to acute coronary syndrome (ACS). He was in shock and had to be put on inotropes and assisted ventilation. He too had bled earlier from esophageal varices and he had a low platelet count of 60,000/mL. He had undergone CAG previously that revealed a three-vessel disease. He was counseled then to consider either a coronary artery bypass grafting (CABG) or angioplasty with a very high risk of periprocedure mortality. In view of the inherent high risk, neither the patient nor the treating physicians were keen on any interventional procedure.

> However, the present situation was different and it involved life or certain death. The author did coronary angiography which revealed total mid-RCA occlusion and near total ostial circumflex lesion besides earlier left main left anterior descending artery (LAD) lesion. Keeping in mind the treatment dilemmas and challenges in such a situation, the author decided to perform balloon angioplasty of the RCA lesion and also the ostial lesion in left circumflex artery. The author could do away with aggressive antiplatelet therapy. Fortunately, there was immediate and satisfactory reperfusion of the myocardium with TIMI III flow and a nonsignificant dissection. This patient's general condition improved dramatically—allowing me to discharge him from the hospital during the next couple of days.

ASSOCIATION BETWEEN LIVER CIRRHOSIS AND CORONARY ARTERY DISEASE

It has been widely reported that heart and liver interact and affect each other. However, causality between liver cirrhosis and coronary artery disease (CAD) is uncertain.[1,2] Earlier, liver disease was thought to have a protective effect against CAD.[3,4] Some of the autopsy studies done in mid-20th century fed this speculation. These autopsy studies revealed reduced incidence of cardiovascular atherosclerosis and myocardial infarction in the cadavers with portal cirrhosis.[4,5] On the contrary, recent literature reveals increased incidence of CAD, varying from 2.5% to 25%, among the patients enlisted for liver transplantation.[6-9] It is interesting to note however that these studies differed in the manner in which CAD was defined. Controls in these studies were inadequate. These studies adopted different diagnostic parameters. Also, these studies involved different individuals in terms of cardiac symptoms and history. As a result, there is a limited understanding of the prevalence of anatomically confirmed CAD in the patients with liver cirrhosis at present. Mortality and morbidity in cirrhotic patients, especially after a major surgery such as liver transplantation, are unfavorably influenced if these patients have an underlying CAD. Majority of the nongraft-related deaths after liver transplantation are attributed to cardiovascular complications.[10-12] Therefore, assessment of cardiovascular risk and prevention of CAD are of utmost importance to prevent death under normal conditions and during perioperative period in patients with liver cirrhosis.

An et al. conducted a major study to assess prevalence of silent CAD in cirrhotic patients. They enrolled cirrhotic patients who had neither the history nor symptoms of heart disease in an ongoing patient registry. All of these patients underwent coronary computed tomography (CT) angiography as part of cardiac evaluation before liver transplantation surgery. An et al. compared the results of this subgroup with matched individuals in nonhepatic population.[1] They found that prevalence of CAD among the nonsymptomatic patients with liver cirrhosis did not differ from the prevalence among propensity score-matched nonhepatic group however nonobstructive CAD was more prevalent in cirrhotics (Fig. 1).

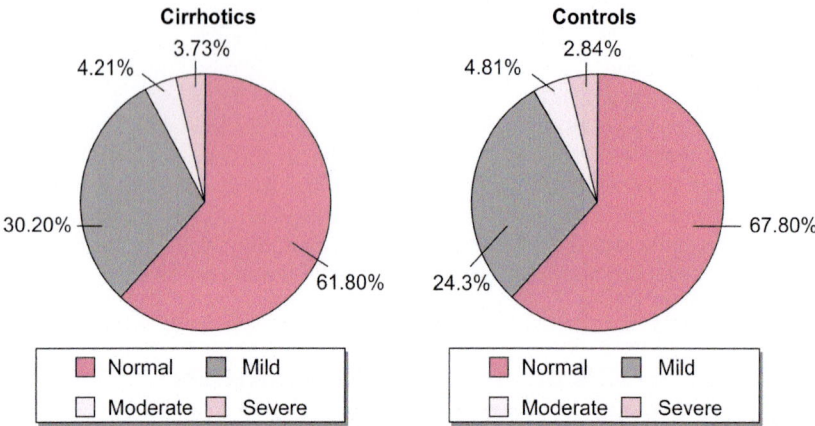

FIG. 1: Distribution of coronary artery stenosis on coronary computed tomography angiography among all cirrhotics (n = 1,045) and controls (n = 6,283). The prevalence of significant obstructive coronary artery disease (CAD) was similar in the two groups [7.9% (83/1,045) vs. 7.7% (486/6,283); p = 0.803], in contrast to that of mild nonobstructive CAD [30.2% (316/1,045) vs. 24.4% (1532/6,283); p <0.001].

Another multivariable analysis found that prevalence of CAD was independent of clinical parameters that can be affected by the severity of liver cirrhosis such as hyperlipidemia, arterial hypertension, diabetes mellitus and body mass index (BMI).[13-17] However, cirrhotic patients had a greater risk for nonobstructive heart lesions which have a more favorable course.[18-22] Prevalence of obstructive CAD in both sets of population was 8% and the traditional risk factors such as age, sex, hypertension and diabetes contributed substantially toward the narrowed coronary arteries in hepatic patients. In this study, patients with liver cirrhosis had more extensive involvement of the coronary arteries compared to noncirrhotic patients and this was regardless of the severity of atherosclerosis. However, this effect did not reach statistical significance for obstructive CAD in the matched sample.

A study by Yong et al. reported a higher mortality after liver transplant in patients with multivessel disease and it was independent of severity of coronary stenosis.[23] It is important to remember that multivessel disease is an important predictor of cardiovascular events in obstructive as well nonobstructive lesions.[20-22]

Moderate-to-severe CAD is found in the candidates for liver transplantation—amounting to 27% of the candidates in some of the recent studies.[6,7,9] These findings suggest that cirrhotic conditions promote CAD. The following epidemiological notions led the authors of these studies to draw their conclusions:
- Approximately half of the patients with nonalcoholic fatty liver disease (NAFLD) including silent or burnt-out steatohepatitis meet the diagnostic

criteria for metabolic syndrome and subsequently have an increased risk of ischemic heart disease
- Thanks to the advances in medical care, patients with liver transplant survive longer[8,14] and putative cardiopathological predictors such as age, sex, hypertension and diabetes are strongly associated with CAD.[1]

Diabetes mellitus is one of the atherosclerogenic factors which is not infrequently detected in many patients with hepatopathy.[6,7,9,24] In addition, long-standing diabetes is usually followed by cirrhosis in many instances. It may be because alcohol consumption and defects of carbohydrate metabolism are the pathogenic factors common to both these conditions. However, it is debatable whether diabetes is more atherogenic when compared to cirrhosis.[24] The findings of these studies have led to the recommendations that assiduous control of blood sugar and screening for occult CAD must be paid attention to in patients with cirrhosis and diabetes. Many recent studies have concluded that heavy and binge drinking of alcohol carries greater risk for CAD when compared to light-moderate drinking.[25,26]

ASSOCIATION OF HEPATITIS C VIRUS INFECTION AND CORONARY ARTERY DISEASE

A study by Ashraf et al. tried to assess subclinical atherosclerosis by measuring carotid intima-media thickness (CIMT) and epicardial fat thickness (EpFT). They found statistically significant increase in both these parameters in patients with cirrhosis due to hepatitis C. In comparison to this group, the control group as well as noncirrhotic patents of hepatitis C had smaller CIMT and EpFT.[27] These findings reveal that patients with hepatitis C are more likely to harbor subclinical atherosclerosis especially when it proceeds to cirrhosis. A study by Butt et al. agrees with this study. Their study found a higher risk of atherosclerosis and CAD in patients with hepatitis C virus (HCV) infection after adjustment for traditional risk factors.[28] Yet another study by Romero-Gómez revealed a strong link between HCV infection and atherogenic process. Their study revealed a link between HCV infection and risk of CAD, carotid atherosclerosis, peripheral vascular disease and finally cardiovascular disease-related mortality.[29]

Some studies have revealed that HCV infection is an independent risk for carotid atherosclerosis.[30,31] However, the findings of some other studies are contrary to the above mentioned studies. A study has shown that chronic viral hepatitis may protect from atherosclerosis in the carotid arteries.[32] Similarly no independent association was found between serological markers for hepatitis C infection and cardiovascular morbidity and atherosclerosis in carotid arteries in another report.[33]

ACUTE CORONARY SYNDROME AND LIVER CIRRHOSIS

In the study by Lin et al. of 57,214 cirrhosis patients, incidence rates of ACS and peripheral arterial disease (PAD) were 2.81 and 2.97 per 1,000 person-years, respectively.[34] ACS was more prevalent in cirrhotic cohort risk being highest among members of the cirrhosis cohort with ascites. This study suggested that cirrhosis predisposes to ACS.

CORONARY ARTERY DISEASE AND NONALCOHOLIC FATTY LIVER DISEASE

Nonalcoholic fatty disease of the liver is considered as the hepatic manifestation of "metabolic syndrome". It is one of the common liver disorders in the industrialized world and it is associated with a significantly increased risk for CAD.[35-37] On conventional ultrasound, increased incidence of nonalcoholic steatohepatitis (NASH) was found in patients who underwent coronary angiography and in whom CAD was subsequently detected.[38] NAFLD is defined as lipid accumulation in more than 5% of the hepatocytes in liver histology.

Coronary artery disease and NAFLD share common risk factors—metabolic syndrome being the most common of these. NAFLD is particularly common among diabetic patients and it is associated with increased risk for CAD when compared to general population.[37] Even though NAFLD is not directly linked to increased mortality, it is an important risk factor for subsequent development of NASH. As much as 10–30% of the patients with NAFLD develop NASH and a third of these progresses to liver cirrhosis with its well-known detrimental effects—including hepatocellular carcinoma (HCC).

Friedrich-Rust et al. detected high incidence of NAFLD (72.7%) in patients undergoing coronary angiography.[35] In this study, patients with severe CAD had higher degree of hepatic steatosis when compared to patients with minor or no CAD. Wong et al. reported similar findings.[38]

A study by Lin et al. included 57,214 patients from Taiwan National Health Insurance claims data with a diagnosis of cirrhosis during the period between 2000 and 2010. In this study, the overall incidence rates of ACS and PAD were 2.81 and 2.97 per 1,000 person-years, respectively, in the cirrhosis cohort. The risk of ACS was higher in the cirrhosis cohort. The risk of ACS was even higher in cirrhotic patients who had ascites. This study concluded that ACS and PAD were more commonly associated with chronic liver disease and cirrhosis when compared to patients without liver disease.

PERCUTANEOUS CORONARY INTERVENTION IN END-STAGE LIVER DISEASE

The available statistics about the prevalence of CAD in cirrhotic patients are sketchy and often contradictory. Some of the older figures based on autopsy and liver transplant studies reveal that less than 1% of the patients with liver cirrhosis harbor concurrent CAD. However, more recent studies report a much higher prevalence ranging between 2.7% and 30%. The highest percentage of CAD prevalence is reported in cirrhotic patients under evaluation for liver transplant.[1,39] As a result, available guidelines for management of CAD in liver cirrhosis are scanty. According to a 2005 guideline by the AHA/ACC/SCAI, dual antiplatelet therapy (DAPT) along with clopidogrel should be used for at least 12 months after a successful percutaneous coronary intervention (PCI).[40] Hemorrhage is the most dreaded complication of DAPT in the setting of cirrhosis. Majority of the bleeding episodes come from the gastrointestinal (GI) tract.[41,42] A proposed hypothesis for pathogenesis of GI hemorrhage is that irreversible inhibition of cyclooxygenase-1 (COX-1) enzyme by aspirin leads to vasoconstriction and decreased mucus secretion in the GI mucosa leaving it vulnerable for injury.[43] Some of the studies have reported significant reduction of prostaglandin levels in rectal, duodenal and gastric mucous membrane.[44] Some double-blind, placebo-controlled studies have reported that 1-4% of the cirrhotic patients undergoing PCI suffer at least one such episode of GI bleed.[45-47] Advanced age along with history of peptic ulcer, usage of nonsteroidal anti-inflammatory drug (NSAID) and anticoagulants are some of the risk factors for bleeding episodes in GI tract after PCI. The current recommendations to prevent GI bleed in cirrhotic patient in post-PCI setting include prescription of proton-pump inhibitor therapy in patients with history of peptic ulcer disease and eradication of *Helicobacter pylori* infection if present.[48] Management of GI bleeding after PCI includes a delicate balancing between risk of in-stent thrombosis and further episodes of life-threatening hemorrhage. The cirrhotic patients are particularly vulnerable for GI bleed because it is reported that at least half of these patients have GI varices at the time of presentation and 8% of them develop varices subsequently.[7] Blood stasis in the portal veins results in increased pressure leading to development of extrahepatic, portosystemic shunts.[8]

A retrospective analysis of 1,218 patients by Alazzawi et al. revealed that cirrhotic patients undergoing PCI have unfavorable outcomes. This study reported a five-time increased risk of in-hospital death in cirrhotic patients when compared to noncirrhotic patients.[49] Patients with cirrhosis had a greater chance of GI bleed—requiring frequent blood transfusions. In this study, as much as 73% of the bleeding events were from upper GI tract with a higher mortality when compared to 27% of the patients who bled from the lower GI tract.

Singh et al. collected data from nationwide sample during the period between 2005 and 2012.[50] They identified reperfusion therapy (PCI) offered to the patients with established cirrhosis. Out of the 1,051,242 PCIs performed during the study period, 122,342 were done on patients with cirrhosis. A propensity-matched analysis revealed a two times higher mortality when bare-metal stents were used instead of drug-eluting stents. This study concludes that even though it is riskier when compared to noncirrhotic general population, PCI continues to be a safe and plausible option for reperfusion of myocardium in patients with liver cirrhosis. The study recommends use of drug-eluting stents instead of bare-metal stents.

■ CORONARY ARTERY BYPASS GRAFTING SURGERY IN PATIENTS WITH LIVER CIRRHOSIS

In the past two decades, remarkable advancements have taken place in medical management and life expectancy of the patients with cirrhosis. This in turn has increased the eligibility of the cirrhotic patients for major cardiac surgery. Following are the recent advancements in medical management of liver cirrhosis:
- Introduction of prophylactic β-blockers to decrease portal hypertension
- Widespread application of endoscopic modalities to treat esophageal varices
- Availability of transjugular intrahepatic portosystemic shunts (TIPS)
- Spontaneous bacterial peritonitis prophylaxis
- Effective medications to suppress hepatitis viral replication.

The above-mentioned advancements have increased the life expectancy in the patients with end-stage liver disease (ESLD). Since the patients with ESLD are living longer, HCC (complication of cirrhosis) and CAD have become more common in this group of patients. The severity of liver disease contributes directly to the overall morbidity and mortality from cardiac surgery. The Child-Turcotte-Pugh (CTP) classification has been a widely followed evaluation method for patients with cirrhosis of liver.[51] CTP was developed initially to predict surgical mortality after portacaval shunting. Presently, this classification is a disease severity index that assigns points to five different parameters of liver function. These five parameters are: (1) serum bilirubin, (2) albumin, (3) prothrombin time (PT), (4) ascites and (5) encephalopathy. This classification based of five parameters of liver function creates three functional classes of cirrhosis: (1) A, (2) B and (3) C. This method of severity assessment has been shown to correlate with 1-year survival and major postoperative complications after cardiac surgery. Suman et al. found in their analysis that hepatic decompensation and mortality correlated significantly to CTP class and CTP score. A CTP score of >7 emerged as a sensitive predictor of postoperative mortality. This score has a sensitivity of 86%, specificity of 92%, and negative predictive value of 97% and positive predictive value of 67%, respectively.[52]

In the setting of liver cirrhosis, the physiologic challenge of cardiac surgery is tolerated poorly. The usual risks associated with any major cardiac surgery are amplified when there is a concomitant severe liver disease. The risks associated with anesthesia, transfusion of large volumes, coagulopathy and disseminated intravascular coagulation (DIC) tend to be amplified in patients with liver cirrhosis. However, the principal elements of hepatic injury are physiological stress of hypotension, hypoperfusion and ischemia-reperfusion. The cardiopulmonary bypass (CPB) employed during a major cardiac surgery imposes physiologic, immunologic and metabolic demands on the liver. Nonpulsatile flow, decreased cardiac output, and hypotension constitute the principal parameters of CPB. The hepatic perfusion is decreased by as much as 20% and hepatic arterial blood flow is reduced by 20–45% through vasoconstriction at the initiation of CPB. This is a result of increased levels of endogenous catecholamines.

It is intuitive to avoid cardiac surgery, if possible, in the presence of an advanced liver disease. Potential mortality and morbidity can be minimized by optimizing medical management, lifestyle modification to decrease risk and emphasizing percutaneous procedures like TIPS.

■ ANTIPLATELET TREATMENT AFTER STENT IMPLANTATION IN LIVER DISEASE

The vexed issue of antiplatelet therapy after PCI in cirrhotic patients is confounded by a lack of large randomized trials. Present treatment regimens are based on a few small observational studies. A retrospective analysis by Russo et al. studied complications in cirrhotic patients who received a coronary stent followed by clopidogrel and aspirin.[53] They compared cirrhotics with stents with an age- and sex-matched control group of cirrhotic patients without stents and not on aspirin. This study included 423 patients of liver cirrhosis who were subjected to evaluation for liver transplantation. Sixteen of these patients (3.8%) received a stent and nine of them underwent liver transplantation subsequently. Two of the patients who received stent suffered a fatal bleeding from the GI varices while two from the control group had a nonfatal variceal bleed during follow-up period and while on antiplatelet therapy. There were no significant differences in the requirement for blood transfusions between the nine patients of liver transplantation and the control group. This study found coronary stenting followed by antiplatelet therapy safe in cirrhotic patients without varices. They also found the coronary stents safe if the cirrhotic patients are probable candidates for liver transplant.[53]

Another study by Krill et al. concludes that DAPT need not be withheld for fear of GI bleed in cirrhotic patients subjected to PCI. Their study encourages use of proton-pump inhibitors.

As regard to platelet count as has been elaborately discussed elsewhere in the book, DAPT can be safely administered if platelet count is above 30,000/mL and aspirin alone definitely if count is above 20,000/mL and possibly if above 10,000/mL.

■ BETA-BLOCKERS IN ACUTE MYOCARDIAL INFARCTION WITH CIRRHOSIS

One of the dreaded complications in patients with cirrhosis and ESLD is possibility of fatal hemorrhage from the GI varices. As much as half of the cirrhotic patients have varices and one-third of these patients are likely to bleed. The reported mortality due to variceal bleeding is 50% during the initial episode and 30% during subsequent bleeding incidents. In view of the much feared complication of GI bleed, a frantic search is on for an effective medication to prevent such bleeding events. Introduction of nonselective β-blockers by Lebrec and colleagues in the 1980s was found effective for secondary as well as primary prevention of GI hemorrhage in cirrhotic patients.[54,55] Mechanism of action of nonselective β-blockers in preventing GI bleed is two-fold. Firstly, it puts a halt to the rising heart rate. Secondly, it reduces pressure in the portal veins by decreasing blood flow in the splanchnic circulation.[56] A study has found the β1-selective blockers less effective when compared to nonselective β-blockers in the management of portal hypertension in cirrhotic patients.[57,58]

Coexistence of myocardial infarction in liver cirrhosis poses a difficult challenge to the treating physician. The literature on cardiovascular subjects has so far revealed that β1-selective blockers are effective in many conditions such as CAD, heart failure and acute myocardial infarction (AMI). This set of drugs is thought to regulate heart rate with fewer side effects. Therefore, in the event of AMI in cirrhotic patients, the conflicting choice between nonselective and β1-selective blockers becomes inevitable.

Wu et al. tried to find a definitive answer to this dilemma through their study.[59] They retrieved medical records from the National Health Insurance Research Database (NHIRD) of Taiwan during 2001–2013. They enrolled a total of 203,995 patients with AMI—6,355 of these patients had concurrent liver cirrhosis. A propensity score matching of the patients on β-blockers was done. The 218 patients on β1-selective blockers and an equal number (218) of patients on nonselective β-blockers were studied during a 2-year follow-up. This study found that patients on β1-selective blockers had significantly fewer cardiac and cerebrovascular events. This finding showed a trend toward lower all-cause mortality and nonworsening liver outcome.

The study by Wu et al. was the first one to prove that β1-selective blockers are beneficial in patients with cirrhosis. Their finding is contrary to the existing belief that only the nonselective blockers are beneficial in the setting of AMI with concurrent liver cirrhosis.

■ CORONARY ARTERY DISEASE AND ORTHOTOPIC LIVER TRANSPLANT

Patients scheduled for orthotopic liver transplantation (OLT) typically undergo an extensive preoperative cardiac evaluation. Patients with ESLD are at greater risk than the general population for CAD, and up to 25% of these patients might have subclinical CAD. Investigators have questioned whether current practices are effective in diagnosing underlying CAD in OLT patients. The cardiac-cause mortality rate in patients with liver disease and CAD exceeds 40%. The American Association for the Study of Liver Diseases recommends that dobutamine stress echocardiography (DSE) be performed in patients who will undergo OLT, and the American College of Cardiology recommends against invasive testing; however, investigators in several cohort studies have noted that the sensitivity and specificity of DSE can be influenced by the hyperdynamic and vasodilatory states in such patients. In cirrhotic patients, DSE has poor sensitivity and specificity. Snipelisky et al. reviewed the electronic medical records of 2,010 patients who underwent OLT in their hospital from 2000 through 2010. The 51 patients who had undergone invasive coronary angiography were selected for the study and were classified to have mild CAD (<50% stenosis of a major coronary artery), moderate CAD (50–70% stenosis), or severe CAD (>70% stenosis). They determined whether CABG or PCI with stent placement had been performed within 6 months before OLT. They found that the patients who underwent intervention before OLT were at high risk for cardiac-cause death. All the patients who died of a cardiac cause had undergone PCI or CABG before OLT. They concluded that, despite coronary intervention, mortality rates remain high in OLT patients who have severe CAD.

Epilogue

- Coronary artery disease is widely prevalent in patients with liver cirrhosis both overt and silent
- Multivessel coronary disease is a major predictor of mortality during liver transplantation
- Acute coronary syndrome is more prevalent in cirrhotic cohorts especially those with ascites
- Coronary artery bypass grafting preferably be avoided in advanced liver disease
- Percutaneous coronary intervention is relatively safer option compared with CABG in advanced liver disease and should be undertaken whenever indicated especially when liver transplant is planned
- In desperate situations, drug-eluting stents may be used in PCI patients with liver cirrhosis and DAPT may be employed even with history of varices as long as platelet count is above 30,000/mL
- Proton-pump inhibitors should be routinely administered to prevent GI bleeding
- It is unclear whether coronary intervention (PCI or CABG) will improve survival after liver transplantation in those with severe CAD.

REFERENCES

1. An J, Shim JH, Kim SO, et al. Prevalence and prediction of coronary artery disease in patients with liver cirrhosis: a registry-based matched case-control study. Circulation. 2014;130:1353-62.
2. Møller S, Bernardi M. Interactions of the heart and the liver. Eur Heart J. 2013;34:2804-11.
3. Vaněcek R. Atherosclerosis and cirrhosis of the liver. Bull World Health Organ. 1976;53: 567-70.
4. Howell WL, Manion WC. The low incidence of myocardial infarction in patients with portal cirrhosis of the liver: a review of 639 cases of cirrhosis of the liver from 17,731 autopsies. Am Heart J. 1960;60:341-4.
5. Creed DL, Baird WF, Fisher ER. The severity of aortic arteriosclerosis in certain diseases; a necropsy study. Am J Med Sci. 1955;230:385-91.
6. Carey WD, Dumot JA, Pimentel RR, et al. The prevalence of coronary artery disease in liver transplant candidates over age 50. Transplantation. 1995;59:859-64.
7. Kalaitzakis E, Rosengren A, Skommevik T, et al. Coronary artery disease in patients with liver cirrhosis. Dig Dis Sci. 2010;55:467-75.
8. Keeffe BG, Valantine H, Keeffe EB. Detection and treatment of coronary artery disease in liver transplant candidates. Liver Transpl. 2001;7:755-61.
9. Tiukinhoy-Laing SD, Rossi JS, Bayram M, et al. Cardiac hemodynamic and coronary angiographic characteristics of patients being evaluated for liver transplantation. Am J Cardiol. 2006;98:178-81.
10. Mandell MS, Lindenfeld J, Tsou MY, et al. Cardiac evaluation of liver transplant candidates. World J Gastroenterol. 2008;14:3445-51.
11. Therapondos G, Flapan AD, Plevris JN, et al. Cardiac morbidity and mortality related to orthotopic liver transplantation. Liver Transpl. 2004;10:1441-53.
12. Fouad TR, Abdel-Razek WM, Burak KW, et al. Prediction of cardiac complications after liver transplantation. Transplantation. 2009;87:763-70.
13. Campillo B, Richardet JP, Bories PN. Validation of body mass index for the diagnosis of malnutrition in patients with liver cirrhosis. Gastroenterol Clin Biol. 2006;30:1137-43.
14. Targher G, Day CP, Bonora E. Risk of cardiovascular disease in patients with nonalcoholic fatty liver disease. N Engl J Med. 2010;363:1341-50.
15. Dumitraşcu DL, Stanciu L, Dumitraşcu D, et al. The prognostic significance of arterial blood pressure in liver cirrhosis. Rom J Intern Med. 1995;33:155-9.
16. Minuk GY, MacCannell KL. Is the hypotension of cirrhosis a GABA mediated process? Hepatology. 1988;8:73-7.
17. Wlazlo N, Beijers HJ, Schoon EJ, et al. High prevalence of diabetes mellitus in patients with liver cirrhosis. Diabet Med. 2010;27:1308-11.
18. Lin FY, Shaw LJ, Dunning AM, et al. Mortality risk in symptomatic patients with nonobstructive coronary artery disease: a prospective 2-center study of 2,583 patients undergoing 64-detector row coronary computed tomographic angiography. J Am Coll Cardiol. 2011;58:510-9.
19. Leipsic J, Taylor CM, Grunau G, et al. Cardiovascular risk among stable individuals suspected of having coronary artery disease with no modifiable risk factors: results from an international multicenter study of 5,262 patients. Radiology. 2013;267: 718-26.
20. Bittencourt MS, Hulten E, Ghoshhajra B, et al. Prognostic value of nonobstructive and obstructive coronary artery disease detected by coronary computed tomography angiography to identify cardiovascular events. Circ Cardiovasc Imaging. 2014;7:282-91.
21. Min JK, Shaw LJ, Devereux RB, et al. Prognostic value of multidetector coronary computed tomographic angiography for prediction of all-cause mortality. J Am Coll Cardiol. 2007;50:1161-70.

22. Ostrom MP, Gopal A, Ahmadi N, et al. Mortality incidence and the severity of coronary atherosclerosis assessed by computed tomography angiography. J Am Coll Cardiol. 2008;52:1335-43.
23. Yong CM, Sharma M, Ochoa V, et al. Multivessel coronary artery disease predicts mortality, length of stay, and pressor requirements after liver transplantation. Liver Transpl. 2010;16:1242-8.
24. Marchesini G, Ronchi M, Forlani G, et al. Cardiovascular disease in cirrhosis—a point prevalence study in relation to glucose tolerance. Am J Gastroenterol. 1999;94:655-62.
25. Malyutina S, Bobak M, Kurilovitch S, et al. Relation between heavy and binge drinking and all-cause and cardiovascular mortality in Novosibirsk, Russia: a prospective cohort study. Lancet. 2002;360:1448-54.
26. Pearson TA. Alcohol and heart disease. Circulation. 1996;94:3023-5.
27. El-Khalik Barakat AA, Nasr FM, Metwaly AA, et al. Atherosclerosis in chronic hepatitis C virus patients with and without liver cirrhosis. Egypt Heart J. 2017;69:139-47.
28. Butt AA, Xiaoqiang W, Budoff M, et al. Hepatitis C virus infection and the risk of coronary disease. Clin Infect Dis. 2009;49:225-32.
29. Ampuero J, Romero-Gómez M. Assessing cardiovascular risk in hepatitis C: an unmet need. World J Hepatol. 2015;7(19):2214-9.
30. Ishizaka N, Ishizaka Y, Takahashi E. Association between hepatitis C virus seropositivity, carotid-artery plaque, and intima-media thickening. Lancet. 2002;359:133-5.
31. Ishizaka N, Ishizaka Y, Takahashi E. Increased prevalence of carotid atherosclerosis in hepatitis B virus carriers. Circulation. 2002;105:1028-30.
32. Bilora F, Rinaldi R, Boccioletti V. Chronic viral hepatitis: a prospective factor against atherosclerosis. A study with echo-color Doppler of the carotid and femoral arteries and the abdominal aorta. Gastroenterol Clin Biol. 2002;26:1001-4.
33. Volzke H, Schwahn C, Wolff B. Hepatitis B and C virus infection and the risk of atherosclerosis in a general population. Atherosclerosis. 2004;174:99-103.
34. Lin SY, Lin CL, Lin CC, et al. Risk of acute coronary syndrome and peripheral arterial disease in chronic liver disease and cirrhosis: a nationwide population-based study. Atherosclerosis. 2018;270:154-9.
35. Friedrich-Rust M, Schoelzel F, Maier S, et al. Severity of coronary artery disease is associated with non-alcoholic fatty liver disease: a single-blinded prospective mono-centre study. PLoS One. 2017;12(10):e0186720.
36. Bang KB, Cho YK. Comorbidities and metabolic derangement of NAFLD. J Lifestyle Med. 2015;5(1):7-13.
37. Musso G, Gambino R, Cassader M, et al. Meta-analysis: natural history of non-alcoholic fatty liver disease (NAFLD) and diagnostic accuracy of non-invasive tests for liver disease severity. Ann Med. 2011;43(8):617-49.
38. Wong VW, Wong GL, Yip GW, et al. Coronary artery disease and cardiovascular outcomes in patients with non-alcoholic fatty liver disease. Gut. 2011;60(12):1721-7.
39. Cichoz-Lach H, Celiński K, Słomka M, et al. Pathophysiology of portal hypertension. J Physiol Pharmacol. 2008;59:231-8.
40. King SB 3rd, Smith SC Jr, Hirshfeld JW Jr, et al. 2007 focused update of the ACC/AHA/SCAI 2005 guideline update for percutaneous coronary intervention: a report of the American College of Cardiology/American Heart Association Task Force on Practice Guidelines. J Am Coll Cardiol. 2008;51:172-209.
41. Tanigawa T, Watanabe T, Nadatani Y, et al. Gastrointestinal bleeding after percutaneous coronary intervention. Digestion. 2011;83:153-60.
42. Kauffman G. Aspirin-induced gastric mucosal injury: lessons learned from animal models. Gastroenterology. 1989;96:606-14.
43. Cryer B, Feldman M. Effects of very low dose daily, long-term aspirin therapy on gastric, duodenal, and rectal prostaglandin levels and on mucosal injury in healthy humans. Gastroenterology. 1999;117:17-25.

44. Hallas J, Dall M, Andries A, et al. Use of single and combined antithrombotic therapy and risk of serious upper gastrointestinal bleeding: population based case-control study. BMJ. 2006;333:726.
45. Nikolsky E, Stone GW, Kirtane AJ, et al. Gastrointestinal bleeding in patients with acute coronary syndromes: incidence, predictors, and clinical implications: analysis from the ACUITY (Acute Catheterization and Urgent Intervention Triage Strategy) trial. J Am Coll Cardiol. 2009;54:1293-302.
46. Abbas AE, Brodie B, Dixon S, et al. Incidence and prognostic impact of gastrointestinal bleeding after percutaneous coronary intervention for acute myocardial infarction. Am J Cardiol. 2005;96:173-6.
47. Dai X, Makaryus AN, Makaryus JN, et al. Significant gastrointestinal bleeding in patients at risk of coronary stent thrombosis. Rev Cardiovasc Med. 2009;10:14-24.
48. Tan VP, Yan BP, Kiernan TJ, et al. Risk and management of upper gastrointestinal bleeding associated with prolonged dual antiplatelet therapy after percutaneous coronary intervention. Cardiovasc Revasc Med. 2009;10:36-44.
49. Alazzawi Y, Alabboodi Y, Fasullo M, et al. The morbidity and mortality risks following percutaneous coronary interventions in cirrhosis. J Liver. 2017;6:216.
50. Singh V, Patel NJ, Rodriguez AP, et al. Percutaneous coronary intervention in patients with end-stage liver disease. Am J Cardiol. 2016;117(11):1729-34.
51. Child C, Turcotte J. Surgery and portal hypertension, In: Child C (Ed). The Liver and Portal Hypertension, 3rd edition. Philadelphia, PA: WB Saunders; 1964. pp. 50-64.
52. Suman A, Barnes DS, Zein NN, et al. Predicting outcome after cardiac surgery in patients with cirrhosis: a comparison of Child-Pugh and MELD scores. Clin Gastroenterol Hepatol. 2004;2:719-23.
53. Russo MW, Pierson J, Narang T, et al. Coronary artery stents and antiplatelet therapy in patients with cirrhosis. J Clin Gastroenterol. 2011;46:339-44.
54. Lebrec D, Nouel O, Corbic M, et al. Propranolol—a medical treatment for portal hypertension? Lancet. 1980;2:180-2.
55. Lebrec D, Poynard T, Hillon P, et al. Propranolol for prevention of recurrent gastrointestinal bleeding in patients with cirrhosis: a controlled study. N Engl J Med. 1981;305:1371-4.
56. Ge PS, Runyon BA. The changing role of beta-blocker therapy in patients with cirrhosis. J Hepatol. 2014;60:643-53.
57. Hillon P, Lebrec D, Munoz C, et al. Comparison of the effects of a cardioselective and a nonselective beta-blocker on portal hypertension in patients with cirrhosis. Hepatology. 1982;2:528-31.
58. Westaby D, Melia WM, Macdougall BR, et al. Beta-1-selective adrenoreceptor blockade for the long term management of variceal bleeding. A prospective randomised trial to compare oral metoprolol with injection sclerotherapy in cirrhosis. Gut. 1985;26:421-5.
59. Wu VC, Chen SW, Ting PC, et al. Selection of β-blocker in patients with cirrhosis and acute myocardial infarction: a 13-year nationwide population-based study in Asia. J Am Heart Assoc. 2018;7:e008982.

CHAPTER 7

Acute Coronary Syndrome in Hematological Disorders

Prologue
Back from the Brink

Recently, a 54-year-old gentleman, father of a young physician, was referred to me for cardiac evaluation. He experienced occasional chest pain on exertion. His tread-mill-test was strongly positive for inducible ischemia. This led me to proceed with the coronary angiogram (CAG). The CAG revealed a stenotic plaque lesion in the left anterior descending artery (LAD)—occluding almost 90% of the lumen. The patient and his physician son readily agreed for implanting a drug-eluting stent (DES) in the LAD. The angioplasty procedure itself was uneventful. The author gave 5,000 IU of heparin and put the patient on dual antiplatelet therapy (DAPT)—consisting of clopidogrel and aspirin. All was well until it was time to remove the femoral sheath from the groin vessel—3 hours after the procedure as is the standard operating protocol. The moment the femoral sheath was removed, all hell broke loose. There was a continuous hemorrhage from the puncture site in the groin. Usually, the hemorrhage stops 15 minutes to half an hour after the sheath-removal. In this case, there was no sign of cessation of bleeding even 3–4 hours after the sheath was removed. The attending nurse and other staff kept a continuous manual pressure—hoping that bleeding would stop. But, it was not to be. The author was flummoxed. The author thought of calling the vascular surgeon to suture the bleeding femoral artery. However, unexpectedly an idea flashed. The author decided to transfuse fresh-frozen plasma. Lo and behold, the bleeding stopped! That was when it struck me that this patient might be harboring a hitherto undetected bleeding diathesis. On further investigations, he was found to be harboring milder variety of hemophilia which is an inherited bleeding diathesis disorder. Since this gentleman had a milder variety, it remained undiagnosed till now. That is the reason why nothing significant emerged from the medical history till this procedure was undertaken. Subsequently the author had to stop clopidogrel, reduce aspirin dose to minimum as even a minor trauma would cause a bruise or discoloration of the skin. The author shudder to think what could have possibly happened if a minor coronary vessel had ruptured during the procedure. Fortunately, he continues to tolerate 50 mg of aspirin without any major bleeding episode so far and he has not had any major cardiovascular event 2 years down the line. Surely, this incident taught me an important lesson. This patient and the author literally came back from the proverbial brink.

INTRODUCTION

Serious disturbances in blood rheology are reported in many hematological conditions. Many a times, such changes in blood rheology lead to prothrombotic status. The conditions in this group are frequently associated with an imbalance between coagulation and thrombolytic factors leading to systemic inflammation and heightened risk of serious bleeding. The outcomes of various reperfusion therapies such as coronary angioplasty and coronary bypass grafting (CABG) may be altered by occurrence of bleeding in coagulopathies such as hemophilia. Acute coronary syndrome (ACS) is often accompanied by various changes in blood homeostasis.[1]

ACS IN PATIENTS WITH THROMBOCYTOPENIA AND THROMBOTIC THROMBOCYTOPENIC PURPURA

Whenever an atherosclerotic plaque ruptures, platelets play a significant role in the thrombosis and occlusion of coronary arteries.[1] This fact was amply proved even in thrombotic thrombocytopenic purpura (TTP) patients by a large, multi-institutional cohort study in 2013. This study included 4,032 patients from the 2001–2010 Nationwide Inpatient Sample database. All of these patients were diagnosed with TTP and they were treated with plasmapheresis (mean age 47.5 years, 67.7% female). This study showed that despite adequate treatment for TTP, 5.7% of these patients developed an ACS during hospitalization. The predictors of acute myocardial infarction (AMI) included age, tobacco use, known coronary artery disease (CAD) and congestive heart failure (CHF).[2]

ACS IN IMMUNE THROMBOCYTOPENIC PURPURA

Low platelet count is the hallmark of immune thrombocytopenic purpura (ITP). However, it is rarely associated with ACS. Even though ITP is associated with an increased risk of hemorrhage, atherosclerosis and thrombosis are also common in this condition.[3,4]

A review comparing the results of CABG versus percutaneous coronary intervention (PCI) in subjects with ITP was published in 2011. This review included 32 patients of ITP who underwent CABG (mean age 63 ± 10 years) and 15 subjects of ITP who were subjected to PCI (mean age 62 ± 16 years). This study concluded that revascularization methods are safe as well as feasible and that antiplatelet therapy may be stopped once the platelet count slips below 20,000/μL.

Probable etiologies of increased propensity for thrombosis in ITP include:[5]
- Antibody reaction to platelets
- Release of platelet microparticles
- Release of larger and younger platelets
- Splenectomy
- Treatments such as steroids or danazol

- Autoantibodies directed against antigens present on thrombocyte as well as endothelial surface
- Antiphospholipid antibodies.

ACS IN VON WILLEBRAND DISEASE

The von Willebrand factor (vWF) plays an important role in the coagulation cascade. Elevated level of vWF is often associated with increased risk of CAD. As much as 1.5- to 2-fold increase in vWF is reported during first 24 hours after ST elevation myocardial infarction (STEMI) and the levels peak at 48–72 hours.[1] Lim et al. studied ten patients of von Willebrand disease with concomitant ACS. They reported that interventions for revascularization were not complicated by severe hemorrhage in the setting of mild congenital hemorrhagic disease despite the subjects not receiving factor concentrates before coronary angiography. In addition, administration of DAPT for a short duration was tolerated well by these patients. However, patients receiving aspirin for a longer duration had minor bleeding complications but they required monitoring.[6]

Another study with five cases indicated that anticoagulant therapy can be safely administered by giving factor protection when vWF activity levels are maintained at 30%. Martin et al. suggested usage of high-intensity anticoagulation for a short duration during administration of clotting factor. This study recommends maintaining the vWF activity at a level greater than 50% before the interventional procedure.[7]

Hemophilia and Acute Coronary Syndrome

Since the patients with inherited hemorrhagic pathologies have a tendency toward serious bleeding episodes, thrombolysis for MI is not justified. Primary PCI is recommended for STEMI in patients with hemophilia. Bare-metal stents are preferred to DESs. Duration of DAPT can be curtailed to a shorter duration, usually a month, when bare-metal stents are used. It allows rigorous prophylaxis maintaining the factor concentration at 30% or more. In view of the enhanced risk of bleeding, usage of glycoprotein IIb/IIIa inhibitors is not feasible during initial management of STEMI in patients with hemophilia. The activity of the missing clotting factor should be at least 80% at the time of heparin administration and coronary intervention in patients of hemophilia.[8-10]

The ARCHER study in 2015 analyzed the incidence of CVD in hemophilic patients. This study reported 14/1,000 patients for any CVD event, 8.2/1,000 patients for CAD and 3.5/1,000 patients for MI [non-ST elevation myocardial infarction (NSTEMI) and STEMI]. The majority of these patients were treated with revascularization. Out of the 12 patients who underwent revascularization procedures, three underwent CABG while nine underwent PCI. Interventional revascularization was performed with bare-metal stents in six cases while DES was used in one patient. All of the patients who underwent PCI received DAPT for 1–3 months and it was followed by aspirin therapy for longer duration. In addition, prophylactic coagulation factor concentrate was administered to all patients who were subjected to PCI and preoperatively to those who underwent CABG surgery.[11]

Fogarty et al. conducted a 10-year survey of 2,000 hemophiliacs with concomitant ACS. They arrived at two conclusions. Firstly, ACS occurs in younger patients of hemophilia when they have other cardiovascular risk factors. Secondly, secondary prevention cardiovascular prevention and revascularization therapies followed by dual antiplatelet agents are feasible treatment procedures in selected cases.[12]

ACS IN POLYCYTHEMIA VERA AND ESSENTIAL THROMBOCYTHEMIA

Polycythemia vera (PV) is a condition where there is excessive proliferation of red blood cells—causing increase in blood viscosity which in turn results in a tendency toward vascular thrombosis. AMI and heart failure are the main cause of mortality in PV.

Excessive production of platelets is the hall mark of essential thrombocythemia (ET). However, the excessive platelets are dysfunctional leading to increased risk of thrombosis and hemorrhage. In this condition, thromboembolic events are not infrequent—deep vein thrombosis and pulmonary thromboembolism are the common manifestations. AMI is not common in this case.[13]

The ECLAP study recommends low-dose aspirin for the prevention of thromboembolic events and ACS in patients of PV. As per this study, low-dose aspirin reduces the risk of fatal MI by as much as 30% in PV patients.[14] Cytoreductive therapy is a recent addition to the available treatment methods to reduce the risk of thromboembolism in patients of PV. This technique recommends phlebotomy or hydroxyurea in all patients of PV in order to achieve optimal control of blood cell counts.[15] In patients of ET and PV with AMI, prompt percutaneous reperfusion followed by aggressive antithrombotic drug regimen is recommended along with cytoreductive medication. Cytoreductive treatment is linked to an important reduction in the rate of complications due to thrombosis. Hydroxyurea is recommended as a first-line treatment while anagrelide is suggested as a second-line of therapy because of its minimal leukemogenic effects in younger patients.[16]

A retrospective study (2016) recruited 263 patients in order to analyze the rate of AMI in patients with PV and ET. In this study, ten cases of STEMI and four cases of NSTEMI were reported during follow-up period. Majority of the acute coronary events had occurred during the first year after the diagnosis.[17]

AUTOIMMUNE HEMOLYTIC ANEMIA WITH ACUTE MYOCARDIAL INFARCTION

A large Swedish study (2012) conducted a retrospective analysis by enrolling a total number of 336,479 patients admitted between 1987 and 2008 with immune-mediated disease. This study sought to establish connections between immune-mediated diseases including autoimmune hemolytic anemia (AIHA) and atherosclerotic coronary heart disease (CHD). This study indicated a 3.17 [95% confidence interval (CI) 2.16–4.47] risk of CHD in AIHA patients during the first year after hospitalization. However, the established overall risk of CHD for immune-mediated disorders was 2.92 (95% CI 2.84–2.99) in this study.[18]

ACUTE CORONARY SYNDROME IN SICKLE CELL ANEMIA

An autopsy study (2012–2016) of 427 heart specimens from patients who died suddenly reported 12 cases of sickle cell disease (SCD). A retrospective review of the medical history and clinical presentation of these patients revealed that only five of them complained of chest pain. The microscopic examinations showed congested vessels and sickle cell in all the twelve patients. MI with atherosclerosis was found in 41.66% of the heart specimens while MI with normal coronary arteries was found 33.33% of the cases. Myocardial hypertrophy was seen in 8.33% of the cases and media calcification was detected in 16.6 % of the specimens.[19]

CORONARY ARTERY THROMBOSIS IN PATIENTS WITH PAROXYSMAL NOCTURNAL HEMOGLOBINURIA

Intravascular hemolysis followed by hemoglobinuria is the hallmark of paroxysmal nocturnal hemoglobinuria (PNH). It is a rare disorder with a high risk of thrombosis.[20] The pathophysiological mechanism in PNH is characterized by activation of the C5 complement factor through hemoglobin release during hemolysis. It leads to endothelial damage and subsequent intravascular thrombosis. On the other hand, depletion of nitric oxide by circulating hemoglobin molecules leads to arterial thrombosis.

Ziakas et al. reviewed 339 patients with PNH and thrombotic events, with a mean age of 34.5 years. In this study, arterial thrombosis was predominantly seen in coronary arteries leading to MI in younger patients— mean age 35 years. On the contrary, in the older patients, thrombosis caused cerebral strokes. The incidence of MI in this study was relatively low.[21]

ACUTE LEUKEMIA AND THE RISK OF DEVOLOPING ACS

The formation of intravascular thrombi is promoted by two physiopathological pathways. Firstly, increased leukocyte count (hyperleukocytosis) hampers tissue perfusion by altering the blood rheology. This in turn results in affects the microvascular circulation—mostly in central nervous system and respiratory system. The myocardium is affected if there is concomitant atherosclerosis.[22] Secondly, release of potent procoagulant factors from leukemic cells leads to a state of hypercoagulability—resulting in activation of the coagulation cascade and disseminated intravascular coagulation.[23]

A review of 350,000 patients was done from studies published between 1974 and 2005 with the aim of assessing the impact of leukocytosis in patients with ischemic vascular disease. This reviews revealed a significant association between increased white cell count and cardiovascular mortality and morbidity. Leuokocytosis causes microvascular occlusion and enhances the risk of acute thrombosis and accelerates the chronic atherosclerotic process. Therefore, commencement of therapies to reduce white cell count may be appropriate in selected cases. However, hydroxyurea is known to have leukemogenic potential. Therefore administration of hydroxyurea should be confined to high-risk elderly patients and for a short duration.[24]

ACUTE MYOCARDIAL INFARCTION IN HODGKIN'S AND NON-HODGKIN'S LYMPHOMA

In 2007, Anthony et al. followed 7,033 patients registered in the British National Lymphoma Investigation Database from 1967 to 2000. They found that 2,441 patients had died during the follow-up period and that 99.3% of them had a known cause of death. About 166 of these patients had died of MI. The results of the study by Anthony et al. showed that patients of Hodgkin's lymphoma had an increased risk of AMI when compared to general population. It also revealed that relative risk of death due to MI in these patients was more than 2-fold higher. There was a 4-fold increase in the mortality rate due to MI within the first year after the initiation of therapy for Hodgkin's lymphoma. From year 1 to year 14 after initiation of treatment, the relative risk of death increased 2-fold while from year 15 to year 19, risk of death increased 4-fold when compared to general population. This study concluded that mortality risk from MI after initiation of treatment for Hodgkin's lymphoma remains high for the next 25 years. The study concluded further that mortality risk is related directly to supradiaphragmatic radiotherapy, antracycline and vincristine treatment.[25]

MULTIPLE MYELOMA AND MONOCLONAL GAMMOPATHIES

A study by Kristinsson et al. in 2010 using a Swedish database assessed the risk of venous and arterial thrombosis in 18,627 patients with multiple myeloma (MM) and 5,326 patients with monoclonal gammopathy of undetermined significance (MGUS). They discovered that patients of MM as well as MGUS had a heightened risk of arterial and venous thrombosis. The risk of venous thrombosis was more than arterial thrombosis.[26]

PAMI IN IMMUNE THROMBOCYTOPENIC PURPURA

There are two problems associated with treating AMI in patients with concomitant ITP. These are antiplatelet therapy and control of platelet count for prevention of hemorrhage.[27] Bare-metal stent can improve the success rate of PCI in AMI by alleviating the acute occlusion of the coronary arteries. However, the patients treated with metallic coronary stent need DAPT to prevent in-stent thrombosis. The combination of aspirin and thienopyridine derivatives is necessary for minimizing stent thrombosis. Moreover, prolonged DAPT is advocated for patients treated with DESs. Therefore, balloon angioplasty which does not require prolonged DAPT is preferred especially if the reperfusion is optimal and free of dissection.

Bare-metal stent which requires shorter duration of DAPT is next best option. DESs may be reserved in high-risk cases such as diffuse, long lesions, small-sized vessels and poorly controlled diabetes.

The other vexed problem is establishing an optimal platelet count before PCI. Since severe bleeding episodes are uncommon when the platelet count is above 30,000/µL, treatment is initiated only when platelet count slips below 30,000/µL.[28] As long as platelet count remains above 30,000/µL, antiplatelet therapy and heparin can be used with relative safety.[29] Any reperfusion treatment must be considered with extra care and caution when platelet count is <20,000–30,000/µL.[30] Intravenous infusion of gamma-globulin (IVIG) causes rapid increase in platelet count and plasma viscosity. At times, IVIG may induce thromboembolic events including MI during or after infusion.[29] Probable explanation for thromboembolic events after IVIG is the rapid rise of younger and more reactive platelets in response to therapy in patients with concomitant ITP which in turn increases plasma viscosity leading to adverse events. Therefore, due caution is advocated while administering IVIG. The IVIG must be considered only when platelet count is low (<20,000/µL) or when signs of hemorrhage are noticed.

Epilogue

- Coronary artery disease prevalence is fairly common in hematological disorders.
- Hematological disorders with CAD pose a unique challenge with some providing prothrombotic milieu increasing vascular events.
  Some hematological disorders promote bleeding hence creating a situation for interventionalists wanting to use anticoagulation/antiplatelet treatment.
- Despite the challenge involved most of these disorders can be properly managed by PCI or CABG by maintaining optimum clotting factor/platelet levels before intervention in bleeding disorders and using antithrombotic regimen in thrombotic disorders.

REFERENCES

1. Benedek I, Lázár E, Sándor-Kéri J, et al. Acute Coronary Syndromes in Patients with Hematological Disorders. J Cardiovasc Emerg. 2016;2(4):159-68.
2. Balasubramaniyam N, Kolte D, Palaniswamy C, et al. Predictors of in-hospital mortality and acute myocardial infarction in thrombotic thrombocytopenic purpura. Am J Med. 2013;126:1016.e1-7.
3. Frutcher O, Blich M, Jacob G. Fatal acute myocardial infarction during severe thrombocytopenic purpura. Am J Med Sci. 2002;323:279-80.
4. Russo A, Cannizzo M, Ghetti G, et al. Idiopathic thrombocytopenic purpura and coronary artery disease: comparison between coronary artery bypass grafting and percutaneous coronary intervention. Interact Cardiovasc Thorac Surg. 2011;13:153-7.
5. Shen F, Nfor T, Bajwa T. Recurrent acute myocardial infarction in patients with immune thrombocytopenic purpura. J Patient Cent Res Rev. 2014;1:41-5.
6. Lim MY, Pruthi RK. Outcomes of management of acute coronary syndrome in patients with congenital bleeding disorders: a single center experience and review of the literature. Thromb Res. 2012;130:316-22.
7. Martin K, Key NS. How I treat patients with inherited bleeding disorders who need anticoagulant therapy. Blood. 2016;128:178-84.
8. Zawilska K, Podolak-Dawidziak M. Therapeutic problems in elderly patients with hemophilia. Pol Arch Med Wewn. 2012;122:567-76.
9. Staritz P, de Moerloose P, Schutgens R, et al. Applicability of the European Society of Cardiology guidelines on management of acute coronary syndromes to people with haemophilia. Haemophilia. 2013;19:833-40.
10. Fefer P, Gannot S, Lubetsky A. Percutaneous coronary intervention in patients with haemophilia presenting with acute coronary syndrome: an interventional dilemma: case series, review of the literature, and tips for management. J Thromb Thrombolysis. 2013;35:271-8.
11. Minuk L, Jackson S, Iorio A. Cardiovascular disease (CVD) in Canadians with haemophilia: Age-Related CVD in Haemophilia Epidemiological Research (ARCHER study). Haemophilia. 2015;21:736-41.
12. Fogarty PF, Mancuso ME, Kasthuri R, et al. Presentation and management of acute coronary syndromes among adult persons with haemophilia: results of an international, retrospective, 10-year survey. Haemophilia. 2015;21:589-97.
13. Provan D, Baglin T, Dokal I. Oxford Handbook of Clinical Haematology, 4th edition. London: Oxford University Press; 2015. pp. 258-61.
14. Landolfi R, Marchioli R, Kutti J, et al. Efficacy and Safety of Low-Dose Aspirin in Polycythemia Vera. N Engl J Med. 2004;350:114-24.
15. Barbui T, Finazzi G, Falanga A. Myeloproliferative neoplasms and thrombosis. Blood. 2013;122:2176-84.
16. Tortorella G, Calzolari M, Tieghi A, et al. Acute coronary syndrome (ACS) in patients with essential thrombocytemia (ET). What is the best treatment? Int J Cardiol. 2016;203:225-7.
17. Pósfai É, Marton I, Borbényi Z, et al. Myocardial infarction as a thrombotic complication of essential thrombocythemia and polycythemia vera. Anatol J Cardiol. 2016;16:397-402.
18. Zöller B, Li X, Sundquist J, et al. Risk of Subsequent Coronary Heart Disease in Patients Hospitalized for Immune-Mediated Diseases: A Nationwide Follow-Up Study from Sweden. PLoS One. 2012;7:e33442.
19. Bhaskar V, Joshi C. Effect of Sickle Cell Disease on Cardiovascular System: A 4.5 Years Autopsy Study Conducted in a Tertiary Care Center of Central India. Int J Sci Study. 2016;4:188-92.

20. van Bijnen STA, van Heerde WL, Muus P. Mechanisms and clinical implications of thrombosis in paroxysmal nocturnal hemoglobinuria. J Thromb Haemost. 2012; 10:1-10.
21. Ziakas PD, Poulou LS, Rokas GI, et al. Thrombosis in paroxysmal nocturnal hemoglobinuria: sites, risks, outcome. An overview. J Thromb Haemost. 2007;5:642-5.
22. Cohen Y, Amir G, Da'as N, et al. Acute Myocardial Infarction as the Presenting Symptom of Acute Myeloblastic Leukemia With Extreme Hyperleukocytosis. Am J Hematol. 2002;71:47-9.
23. Cahill TJ, Chowdhury O, Myerson SG, et al. Myocardial infarction with intracardiac thrombosis as the presentation of acute promyelocytic leukemia: diagnosis and follow-up by cardiac magnetic resonance imaging. Circulation. 2011;123:e370-2.
24. Coller BS. Leukocytosis and ischemic vascular disease morbidity and mortality: is it time to intervene? Arterioscler Thromb Vasc Biol. 2005;25:658-70.
25. Swerdlow AJ, Higgins CD, Smith P, et al. Myocardial Infarction Mortality Risk After Treatment for Hodgkin Disease: A Collaborative British Cohort Study. J Natl Cancer Inst. 2007;99:206-14.
26. Kristinsson SY, Pfeiffer RM, Björkholm M, et al. Arterial and venous thrombosis in monoclonal gammopathy of undetermined significance and multiple myeloma: a population-based study. Blood. 2010;115:4991-8.
27. Fujino S, Niwa S, Fujioka K, et al. Primary Percutaneous Coronary Intervention by a Stentless Technique for Acute Myocardial Infarction with Idiopathic Thrombocytopenic Purpura: A Case Report and Review of the Literature. Intern Med. 2016;55:147-52.
28. Cines DB, Blanchette VS. Immune thrombocytopenic purpura. N Engl J Med. 2002;346: 995-1008.
29. Zaid G, Dawod S, Rosenschein U. Immune thrombocytopenic purpura and myocardial infarction: a dilemma of management. Isr Med Assoc J. 2013;15:775-6.
30. Liebman HA, Pullarkat V. Diagnosis and management of immune thrombocytopenia in the era of thrombopoietin mimetics. Hematology Am Soc Hematol Educ Program. 2011;2011:384-90.

Acute Coronary Syndrome in Cancer

Choice of Lesser Devil

A 62-year-old mother of a doctor was planning for surgery for recently diagnosed Ca (cancer) colon developed class III angina. Her coronary angiogram showed 90% proximal left anterior descending artery (LAD) lesion. The treatment dilemma was whether surgery for Ca colon first or treatment for coronary artery disease (CAD) first. Surgeon did not want to operate without treating heart lesion before. The cardiac treatment in view of single vessel disease was percutaneous coronary intervention (PCI). However, performing PCI involves dual antiplatelet therapy (DAPT) and deferring gastrointestinal (GI) surgery. Fortunately, surgeon was confident that waiting for a month will not matter for colonic lesion. The author did PCI for LAD using bare-metal stent (BMS). She underwent colonic surgery on aspirin only a month later. Three years later she is nearly cured of Ca colon and repeat coronary angiogram revealed a widely patent bare-metal stent.

A 70-year-old lady with low-grade cerebral astrocytoma presented with ST elevation myocardial infarction (STEMI). She underwent primary PCI as the neurologist assured that astrocytoma does not need any aggressive treatment.

■ INTRODUCTION

Worldwide, cancer and cardiac disease are known to be leading causes of death.[1] There has been a spurt in the number of cancer survivors and concomitant cardiovascular disease thanks to the recent advancements in screening, diagnosis as well as treatment of these conditions. Since there is an overlap of risk factors such as age, smoking, etc. high prevalence of CAD is noticed in patients with a recently diagnosed cancer and in those undergoing active oncologic therapy. Yet another reason for this association is the fact that certain oncologic treatments such as radiation and chemotherapy predispose to early atherosclerosis.[2]

MECHANISMS OF CORONARY ARTERY DISEASE IN CANCER PATIENTS

When compared to general population, there is a significant difference of the mechanism of the CAD and acute coronary syndrome (ACS) in patients with cancer.[3] Secretion of pro inflammatory cytokines is induced by the cancer cells. The cytokines promote endothelial damage—resulting in microvascular permeability for pro coagulating factors such as tissue factor and platelet activating factor.[4] Elevated low-density lipoproteins particles invade the intimal layers of the vessels forming plaques. This chain of events when combined with prothrombotic states in cancer results in overall risk of CAD in cancer patients.[1] In addition, it is observed that endothelium as well as the outer layers of the vessels are damaged by chemotherapy and radiation.

Various chemotherapy drugs affect the coronary arteries in different ways. The 5-FU (5-fluorouracil) causes abnormal vasoreactivity. Paclitaxel and docetaxel cause marked vasospasm leading to ACS. Cisplatin is known cause thrombosis in multiple coronary arteries.[5] Many pathology studies have demonstrated that bleomycin induces endothelial dysfunction, vinblastine causes endothelial apoptosis, while nilotinib and ponatinib induce accelerated atherosclerosis.[6] Prinzmetal angina is known to be triggered by cyclophosphamide while Takotsubo cardiomyopathy—mimicking STEMI, is caused by several chemotherapy agents.[7]

Since ionizing radiation affects the rapidly proliferating noncancerous cells too apart from the cancerous cells, radiotherapy is a known cause of increased risk of ACS due to oxidative stress and inflammation of the endothelial lining of the coronary arteries. Cholesterol plaque formation and thrombosis of the arteries within days after initiation of radiotherapy is demonstrated by pathological studies in animal models. Fibrosis and calcification in all the layers of the vessels is observed after long-term radiation therapy.[8] Abnormal intraplaque hemorrhage after radiation is demonstrated in experimental animal models. This may lead to progression of atherosclerosis, instability of the plaque and subsequently rupture in human atherosclerotic lesions.

There is a multifactorial mechanism for the increased risk of ACS in cancer patients. Increased risk of thrombosis due to coagulation abnormalities caused various malignancies plays an important role in the pathogenesis of STEMI.

ACS PRESENTATION AND MANAGEMENT IN CANCER PATIENTS

Since chemotherapy is known to induce cardiotoxicity resulting in myocardial injury, pre-existing ACS may be worsened by chemotherapy agents. It may complicate presentation of ACS in cancer patients and they may have atypical presentation when compared to general population. Less than one-third of cancer patients with ACS (30.3%) present with chest pain, 44% present with dyspnea and 23% with hypotension.[9] Even though the etiology of the altered pattern of clinical presentation is unclear, probable mechanisms are increased use of analgesics, neurological effects of malignancy itself or the cancer therapy. Therefore, it is wise to screen the cancer patients for ACS whenever they present with uncharacteristic symptoms. An initial diagnosis based on history, risk factors, ECG findings, cardiac biomarkers and other laboratory tests is required. Estimation of the cardiac biomarkers is recommended at the time of presentation and followed by repeat estimation 6 or 8 hours later. Continuous ECG telemetry monitoring is advised along with cardiac biomarkers to exclude other probable causes of chest pain such as pericarditis, Takotsubo cardiomyopathy, etc. Since the cancer patients are usually frail, management of CAD in them is challenging. The challenge is magnified due to the fact that cancer patients tend to have pancytopenia and thrombocytopenia due to aggressive antineoplastic treatment. These impose severe constraints on surgical treatment of solid tumors because the recommended antiplatelet therapy might interfere with the planned surgical interventions. In majority of the cases, conventional treatment of MI with anticoagulants is not feasible.

Many of the patients experiencing myocardial ischemia due to chemotherapy respond favorably once the therapy is suspended temporarily. In addition, administration of calcium channel blockers and oral nitrates are known to relieve symptoms triggered by chemotherapy induced vasospasm with ECG evidence and myocardial ischemia.[10] However, the myocardial ischemia induced by 5-FU is known to recur when the therapy is restarted. The proposed prophylactic treatment with vasodilators does not seem to prevent further episodes of coronary vasospasm and myocardial ischemia.

In all cases of acute STEMI, prompt revascularization therapy with either thrombolytic agents or PCI is recommended for management by the American Heart Association (AHA) and American College of Cardiology (ACC) guidelines. However, these guidelines are difficult to apply in all cases of STEMI in cancer patients. For instance, thrombolytic therapy for acute myocardial infarction is absolutely contraindicated in bleeding disorders such as thrombocytopenia or intracranial malignancy. Similarly, cancer patients are exposed to bleeding diathesis and unacceptable risk of major hemorrhagic events when substantial doses of heparin along with glycoprotein IIB/IIIA inhibitors are given while performing percutaneous intraluminal angioplasty to treat myocardial infarction.

A very low 1-year survival of 26% with conservative management was reported in one of the largest series of 465 cancer patients with cancer and concomitant ACS from a major cancer center.[1] So far, no study is available that compares results of invasive treatment versus conservative management of cancer patients with ACS. However, previously published observational data suggest that STEMI in patients with recent cancer diagnosis (<6 months) treated with PCI carries a 3-fold increased mortality.[11] Moreover, cancer was one of the strongest independent predictors of in-hospital mortality [odds ratio (OR) 3.2] and 1-year mortality (OR 2.15) in cancer patients undergoing PCI. More than 40% increase in cardiovascular morbidity and mortality was observed in large series from Israel, where cancer survivors constituted 7.8% of the total PCIs.[12] No mortality benefit was provided by PCI when compared to conservative medical treatment in a 10-year observation study of 49,515 patients with metastatic cancer and ACS. This study concludes that PCI may not be a preferred option of treatment of patients with metastatic cancer and ACS.[13]

SPECIAL CONSIDERATION OF PERCUTANEOUS CORONARY INTERVENTION PERFORMANCE IN CANCER PATIENTS

Performing PCI in cancer patient with ACS offers a special challenge. Many of these patients already have anemia which can be exaggerated as a consequence of antithrombotic treatment and vascular access leading to excessive bleeding. In turn, it may increase the risk of heart failure as well. Since many malignancies are associated with a hypercoagulable state as a result of reduced fibrinolysis and expression of procoagulant factors, use of antithrombotic agents is essential to prevent ischemic complications. Moreover, since many of the cancer patients need surgical intervention, cessation of antiplatelet therapy increases the risk of in-stent thrombosis. In case of a noncardiac surgery, one of the antiplatelet agents should be continued. Alternatively, short-acting intravenous IIb/IIIa receptor blocker like tirofiban should be initiated just before the scheduled surgery.[14] In some selected cases, balloon angioplasty without stents can be preferred in order to limit the duration of therapy with DAPT. In order to minimize the risk of in-stent thrombosis, BMSs or everolimus-eluting stents must be preferred because of their faster rates of endothelialization.

However, both devices disrupt the endothelial covering of the coronary artery. The stent is re-endothelialized within 8 weeks for BMS and within 1 year for drug-eluting stent (DES). During this time, DAPT is required. Any interruption of DAPT could lead to in-stent thrombosis. This risk could be enhanced by a cancer-related increased tendency for clotting. Therefore, postponement of any surgery is recommended for 6 weeks to 3 months after implantation of BMS and 6–12 months of DES. With chemotherapy, it might be longer, since this could further delay the re-endothelialization of the stent.[15]

In patients with good outcomes and potentially curable malignancy, coronary artery bypass grafting (CABG) may offer advantages over PCI. The fact that prolonged antiplatelet therapy is not required, thereby resulting in lesser bleeding complications, is an additional advantage that CABG offers over percutaneous interventional procedures.[14]

However, in case of a more aggressive type of cancer with a life expectancy of less than a year, PCI is preferred.[14] There is a limited number of published studies concentrating on cancer and outcomes of PCI. Such a scanty data is due to the fact that cancer patients tend to be excluded from the randomized clinical trials of therapies for CAD. In addition, cardiovascular events are underreported in prospective oncological clinical trials. It was reported in a recent study of 3,423 Dutch patients undergoing primary PCI for STEMI from 2006 to 2009 that pre-PCI cancer was associated with increased short-term mortality.[11] The high mortality rate in patients with recently diagnosed cancer contributes to the overall effect of PCI on mortality.[13]

Whenever PCI is indicated BMSs as well as DESs are recommended. However, DESs are preferred because of the lower rate of in-stent thrombosis. Complex coronary lesions like those requiring bifurcation stenting, overlapping stents carry high risk of stent thrombosis and need to be avoided as far as possible. If absolutely indicated then imaging procedures like intravascular ultrasound (IVUS) or optical coherence tomography (OCT) may be utilized to check for stent apposition, adequate expansion which are prevalent in patients with cancer and CAD and are determinants of stent thrombosis.

Cancer is associated with a hypercoagulability state. Along with this, certain specific effects of cancer treatment on hematopoetic cells increase the risk of bleeding.[16] As a result, it is imperative that special attention is required for vascular access while performing PCI. It prevents potential bleeding complications at the vascular access site. Retroperitoneal hemorrhage (RPH), pseudoaneurysm, AV fistula and excessive bleeding are some of the potential complications. Bleeding complications are especially common in patients with thrombocytopenia. It is a good practice to perform assessment of the vascular access site in advance.[17] If there are multiple previous arterial lines, femoral artery should be preferably accessed. Access of radial artery offers easier local hemostasis and greater patient comfort. Radial artery access is preferred whenever a patient is a candidate for both access types.[18]

Thrombocytopenia is another drawback of PCI in cancer patients. Reduced number of platelets is either a manifestation of malignancy or a consequence of chemotherapy.[19] However, if the platelet count is greater than 10,000/µL, prophylactic transfusion of platelets is generally not recommended before cardiac catheterization. However, in case of necrotic tumors, colorectal tumors or melanoma and in whom platelet count drops below 20,000/µL, platelet transfusion should be considered prior to PCI.[20] Platelet transfusion is also recommended whenever the patient has fever, hyperleukocytosis or coagulation abnormality. There is no set minimum level of platelets as a contraindication for coronary angiogram. However, PCI can be performed in cancer patients with thrombocytopenia with a platelet count of more than 30,000/µL after a micropuncture access and suitable attention to hemostasis.[19] The CABG is an option for only those patients with a platelet count of more than 50,000/µL. If the platelet count is more than

10,000/μL, aspirin can be administered to all patients after the PCI according to the guidelines by SCAI. However, P2Y12 agents (clopidogrel, prasugrel) are recommended for only those patients with a platelet count of more than 30,000/μL. Depending on the type of stent used, duration of DAPT therapy can be minimized. Four weeks of DAPT after placing BMS and 6 months after second- or third-generation DESs are recommended.[20]

▪ TREATMENT STRATEGY IN PATIENTS WITH SIMULTANEOUS HEART DISEASE AND CANCER

Treatment Options for Cardiac Disease

Patients who present with both diseases simultaneously pose some extra challenges. The most life-threatening disease should be treated first.[21] Usually, this is heart disease. CAD is the most common heart disease and requires the most attention. To treat CAD, the aim should be to control symptoms, therefore preventing its progression and development into acute coronary syndrome or infarction.[14] The options are medical treatment, PCI without stent, PCI with BMS or with DES, and CABG with or without extracorporeal circulation (ECC). Patients with stable angina can be treated medically and PCI offers no advantages in terms of survival.[14] The choice between PCI and CABG is debatable. A strategy has to take into account the severity of the cardiac disease, the stage of the malignancy and the general condition of the patient. This could determine the choice between PCI and CABG, between a one- or two-stage procedure, and the need for ECC. PCI is preferred if the malignancy is aggressive or widespread. CABG is a good option when the malignancy is potentially curable.[22,23] CABG and cancer surgery can be performed simultaneously as a one- or two-stage procedure.[24] If a two-stage procedure is preferred, a recovery of 4–6 weeks should be anticipated.[25-27] If the tumor is aggressive or rapidly growing, this might compromise long-term survival because a potentially curable disease could become incurable. Hence, the choice between a one- or two-stage approach depends on the stability of cardiac symptoms, the coronary anatomy and the stage of the tumor.[22] For each cardiac treatment option, different types of tumors have to be scrutinized. The three most commonly described malignancies in cardiac patients are from respiratory, digestive and hematological origin. The site of origin has an impact on the surgical treatment strategy and the risk of postoperative infection by contamination. Resection of pulmonary tumors in a small series of 16 patients who recently underwent PCI with a BMS stent demonstrated its safety with the absence of postoperative infarction and cardiac death.[28] Five-year survival was 53%; long-term mortality was mainly due to cancer.

Digestive tract tumors pose different problems. First, digestive tract tumors might be more common in patients with CAD.[29] In patients undergoing colonoscopy, the presence of CAD was identified as an independent predictor for advanced colon carcinoma. This observation[30-32] might be due to common risk factors for both diseases. Second, digestive tract tumors have a bleeding capacity, which complicates matters for the treatment of CAD. Digestive tract tumors have been identified as independent predictors of digestive tract bleeding and clopidogrel increased this risk. If antiplatelet therapy had to be stopped because of digestive bleeding, the cardiac complication rate after PCI increased from 2.4% to 5.8%.[29] For patients with digestive tract tumors, percutaneous coronary angioplasty without stenting could be a temporary solution, but this carries the risk of dissection with acute closure, thrombosis and restenosis. A second PCI with stenting after recovery from cancer surgery might be an alternative, but this option has less predictable results.[14]

■ CARDIAC RISK ASSESSMENT

The cardiologist needs to know what the risks of noncardiac surgery are. First, if the tumor needs emergent surgery, cardiac evaluation should be limited to what is feasible. Second, the stability of CAD needs to be established according to the AHA/ACC guidelines for noncardiac surgery.[33] In the case of significant left main stem or three vessel disease, acute coronary syndrome, unstable angina or infarction, treatment of CAD is needed before cancer surgery. Third, the risk of cancer surgery should be known; breast, endocrine, reconstructive, gynecologic and minor urologic operations are considered low risk; abdominal and urologic operations are considered intermediate risk. Prior PCI/CABG might not be necessary in these patients. In high-risk patients, treatment of CAD by PCI or CABG has priority over the treatment of cancer.[22] Remarkably, in one series of 1,067 patients operated for non-small-cell lung cancer, cardiac comorbidity (mostly CAD) was not identified as a predictor for hospital and long-term outcome after pulmonary resection.[3] This observation could limit the value of cardiac risk assessment. The functional capacity of patients with CAD might provide an indication for invasive cardiac investigation. If a patient is able to walk 100 yards, as has been suggested, a preoperative stress test is not necessary if the cancer surgery has a low-to-intermediate risk.[14] However, a stress test is noninvasive and provides quantitative information concerning exercise tolerance, the response of heart rate, blood pressure and ECG findings. It should be in the clinical routine for most cardiac patients. Cardiac protection can be offered by several drugs: β-blocking agents for controlling heart rate and blood pressure and angiotensin-converting enzyme inhibitors are useful in the case of reduced left ventricular ejection fraction (LVEF). Aspirin, which is an effective platelet inhibitor, should be continued when it has been started earlier.[14]

■ CORONARY ARTERY BYPASS GRAFTING

An important objective of CABG is the reduction of cardiac complications during or after noncardiac surgery.[14] Another objective is symptom relief, provided the anticipated survival for cancer exceeds 6 months, at least for gastric cancer.[26] It remains to be seen whether this statement is also valid for other types of tumors. This limit can be considered short, but it illustrates the importance of the tumor stage in the decision-making process for CABG; CAD seems to not be the limiting factor for survival after surgical treatment. Another useful criterion might be exercise tolerance, which predicts survival in heart patients with cancer.[14] The origin of the tumor can play a role in the treatment strategy. This strategy is influenced by the number of incisions needed and the risk of infections. Pulmonary tumors can be treated simultaneously with heart disease through the same incision, which is not necessarily the case for tumors of the digestive tract. Moreover, risk of contamination and, hence, of mediastinitis, is higher, especially with colon surgery. While it seems more logical to treat pulmonary tumors in a one-stage procedure, this is not necessarily true for tumors of the digestive tract.

Theoretically, PCI could be considered as a first option in patients with gastric cancer. The use of PCI avoids a sternotomy and, hence, the risk of mediastinitis in a one-stage surgical procedure. As an alternative, CABG can be performed with gastrectomy in a second-stage procedure.[26] Moreover, CABG has some advantages: postoperative ischemia and mortality were less compared with patients who underwent PCI[22] and no prolonged DAPT was required after CABG.[14] The CABG should be performed, preferably without ECC. The general condition of the patient and the extent of the tumor also play a role in the treatment strategy. If the patient is in good condition and partial gastrectomy is possible, partial gastrectomy should be performed simultaneously with CABG. If a total gastrectomy is needed, CABG should come first as part of a two-stage procedure. If the patient is in poor condition and the cancer is advanced, a simultaneous procedure is required for oncologic reasons. In patients with early gastric cancer, gastrectomy could be performed once the patient has recovered from CABG.[26] Mediastinitis is a possible complication after a one-stage procedure and should be taken into account, especially when the digestive tract must be opened.[26,27]

In pulmonary tumors, the risk of contamination and, hence, mediastinitis, is less compared with digestive tract tumors and the tumor can often be removed through the same incision. This one-stage procedure has several advantages, such as avoiding:
- Thoracotomy at a later date
- Second surgical trauma
- Delay in treating the malignancy
- Postoperative pain
- Pulmonary dysfunction and atelectasis
- Bleeding and need for transfusion
- Cardiac and renal complications
- Stress and anxiety
- Reducing costs and stay in hospital or intensive care unit.[22,26,27,34-36]

The main disadvantage of a one-stage procedure is a more severe trauma or risk of bleeding.[35] In some cases, several incisions could be needed. A two-stage technique requires an interval in which the patient has the time to recover. This approach is safe with a morbidity and mortality rate lower than a combined procedure (range: 3–10% vs. 5.4–20.8% for mortality and 52% vs. 86% for morbidity).[37-40] The main drawback, however, is the delay of the treatment for cancer, which might result in its progression to an incurable disease. The interval between the operations varied between 7 and 60 days.[22,41,42] The recurrence rate and development of metastasis also varied, but there seemed to be no correlation between the interval and the recurrence rate.[22,41] Although the aforementioned short-term advantages of one-stage procedures are clear, cancer-free survival is the most relevant end point for any combined treatment strategy. It seems that a one-stage approach is beneficial in patients with heart disease and pulmonary tumors. For digestive tract tumors, this is not necessarily the case.

Hematological malignancies, such as chronic lymphocytic leukemia (CLL), are associated with a dysfunctional immunological state. Bleeding, the need for transfusion and the risk of infection, as well as of mortality after cardiac surgery, seemed to be increased in these patients,[34,43-46] but this is not a universal observation.[47] Cardiac surgery did not result in a long-term negative impact on the course of this malignancy. CLL is not a contraindication for heart surgery,[48] but in one series, a high noncardiac long-term mortality was observed.[31] Thrombocytopenia could be the consequence of hematologic malignancies or of their treatment,[2] which should be taken into account.

Heart Disease in Patients with Malignancy in Remission

This section aims to briefly discuss the effects of cancer treatment on the heart and the results of cardiac surgery in those patients previously treated for malignancy. Heart patients who received a previous treatment for cancer with curative intent do not face the difficulties of simultaneous disease. However, some other aspects have to be taken into account. First, the cardiotoxic effects of the previously applied cancer treatment should be added to the classic risk factors of heart disease.[49,50] Second, if such patients require cardiac surgery, specific problems, such as frailty of the internal mammary artery, postoperative sternal infection and the effect of a decreased LVEF on long-term postoperative survival, have to be taken into account.[14,22,30,51]

Chemotherapy has several cardiotoxic effects.[22] The severity of myocardial damage depends on the type of chemotherapy and the type of cellular alterations. Anthracyclines are known for their damaging effects on cardiac myocytes. Several types of damage have been described in detail in extensive reviews. Some types are irreversible, with a lasting effect on the LVEF.[5,49,50,52,53] Fluorouracil, cisplatinum and many other agents cause or worsen CAD.[5,52,53] Antimitotic agents lead to endothelial damage, which in turn leads to atheromatosis. Coronary spasm, thrombophilia and tendency to thrombosis can worsen these effects.[49] Arrhythmias, conduction defects, pericarditis and thromboembolic complications are other side effects of chemotherapy. Radiotherapy of the mediastinum has long-term effects on coronary arteries and on cardiac valves. The incidence of CAD increased by 63% during a median interval of 9 years after radiotherapy.[14,54] This can be the result of fibrosis, fibrointimal hyperplasia, inflammation, reduced nitric oxide synthase, thrombosis, endothelial damage and depletion of smooth muscle cells and endothelial progenitor cells. Typically, there is an ostial stenosis.[30,52,55] Postradiation valve disease is mostly left-sided. Its hallmarks are fibrosis, retraction and calcification. In this progressive condition, regurgitation occurs early and is followed at a later stage by stenosis.

The severity of radiation-induced heart disease and the need for surgical correction depends on the volume of the heart exposed to radiation and the dose received by that volume.[50] Clinical symptoms and signs of radiation valve disease are often underestimated, but at autopsy, findings are documented more often.[55,56] Heart failure, as a consequence of valvular lesions, often needs more than 10 years to become clinically obvious.[57,58] For example, aortic valve stenosis is eight-times more common only 22 years after radiotherapy.[14,54] With improved techniques of radiotherapy, damage to the heart might be reduced.[52,56] Even then, patients who received irradiation of the chest have to be considered as a heterogeneous group, since protocols of radiotherapy depend on the type and stage of the malignancy. In one series, tangential, variable and extensive radiotherapy on the chest were compared for their effect on the outcome after cardiac surgical correction.[59] The malignancies included breast cancer and Hodgkin's and non-Hodgkin's lymphoma. The median interval time between the treatment of malignancy and heart surgery for all groups was well over 10 years (for breast cancer it was 25 years). Hence, it can safely be assumed that cure from malignancy has been obtained for most of these patients. Only for the patients treated with tangential radiotherapy (breast carcinoma) was the postoperative survival near normal, although this group was considerably older than the two other groups. In this group, the cancer mortality was low.[59] In other studies, left- and right-sided radiotherapy for breast cancer were compared for their effect on the heart. No difference could be found up to 10 years,[60,61] but this period might not be enough and subclinical heart disease might go undetected. Moreover, study designs do not allow definitive conclusions to be drawn. Differences in baseline characteristics such as age, comorbid conditions, radiation dose, inclusion of the internal mammary chain[62] and pre-existing heart disease can have an effect of the outcome of heart surgery. However, it is reasonable to assume that reduction of the irradiated cardiac volume, as well as of the radiation dose,[61] reduces the development of heart disease. Deliverance of 25 Gy to the atrium and 30 Gy to the left ventricle resulted in asymptomatic heart disease in patients treated for Hodgkin's disease.[63]

Postoperative sternal infection is uncommon and somewhat comparable for different doses of irradiation. Off-pump CABG is preferable for treating radiation heart disease since irradiated hearts are more vulnerable to ischemia and cooling during ECC.[59]

■ CLINICAL OUTCOME OF CARDIAC PROCEDURES IN PATIENTS WITH CURRENT AND PRIOR MALIGNANCY

Outcome in Patients with Simultaneous Disease

Short-term results of a one-stage procedure are comparable with those after cardiac surgery in patients with prior (and hence supposedly cured) solid tumors: mortality was between 0% and 7.1%, but the series were usually small and included mostly only pulmonary tumors.[25,36,37] Postoperative infections and mortality were higher in patients with CLL, but there would be no effect of cardiac surgery on the course of CLL.[48] In one series, cancer patients had more need for transfusion (80% vs. 49%) or reintubation (8% vs. 0%), pneumonia (15% vs. 6%), sepsis (8% vs. 2%), arrhythmias (42% vs. 34%) and anticoagulation-related complications (7% vs. 0%) compared with controls. Autonomic dysfunction and hypercoagulability by tumoral tissue factor and platelet activation could persist, even after removal of the tumor. An increased infection rate could be related to an increased need for transfusion. Long-term results and quality of life after a one-stage procedure were acceptable. A 5-year survival over 40% can be reached,[36] but the cancer was responsible for most of the long-term mortality.[25] The type and the stage of the tumor played a dominant role, with a drop in 1-year survival from 80% to 50% with advanced cancer.[25,26] The series are too small to draw definitive conclusions. In this respect, the technical possibility to dissect pulmonary lymph nodes during a combined procedure, but without ECC, might be questioned with respect to the effect on survival. The same applies to the surgical exposure of the lower left lobe.[25,36] With an ECC, it is possible to rotate the heart without compromising the circulation and the lower left lobe can be reached more easily, with better long-term survival as a result.[36]

Outcome in Patients with Mainly Prior Malignancy

Patient series with prior malignancy (or series that mix patients with simultaneous and prior malignancies) had varying study designs, which makes comparison of their results difficult. Hospital mortality varied between 2.4% and 13.0%,[43,47,51,57,59] and was within the range of hospital mortality of patients with simultaneous disease. The extent of prior radiotherapy played a major role.[59] Hospital complications of a series including patients with active malignancy, a malignancy in remission or without malignancy were comparable and ranged between 33% and 36%.[43] Long-term survival seemed encouraging with a 5-year survival between 42% and 89%.[47,51,57,59] The interval between treatment of the prior malignancy and cardiac surgery played an important role in postoperative 5- and 10-year survival: the longer the interval, the better the survival. With an interval of 10 years, a normal gender- and age-matched survival had been reached. With shorter intervals or simultaneous disease, death due to metastasis increased.[43,51] Few studies reported independent predictors of survival: a decreased LVEF, presence of chronic obstructive pulmonary disease, presence of cancer or an interval of less than 2 years between treatment of the malignancy have been identified as predictors.[43,51] Symptomatic aortic valve stenosis needs separate consideration since this condition is very life-threatening in the short term. Aortic valve replacement (AVR) is the only life-prolonging and symptom-reducing treatment. Independent predictors of decreased survival after operation were decreased LVEF, concomitant three-vessel disease and presence of cancer.[47] Compared with medical treatment, AVR significantly increased survival (and reached the survival of cancer patients without valve disease), irrespective of cancer status and presence of metastases. Death due to cardiovascular disease occurred only in patients medically treated for calcified aortic valve stenosis. Survival after AVR was only affected by the tumor after 2 years.[47] Although these results point to symptomatic calcified aortic valve stenosis as the more lethal condition in the short term, the latter study shows weaknesses: the decision for surgery seems unclear and it seemed that several patients were unjustly denied AVR because they may have been symptomatic. Moreover, the question of whether operated patients were in better shape compared with unoperated ones remains unanswered.

Prognostic Implications of a Cancer Diagnosis on Outcomes of Patients Undergoing PCI

In a large review of more than 6 million patients who underwent PCI between 2004–2014, Potts et al. identified 1.8% with current diagnosis of cancer and 5.8% with previous history of malignancy.[64] The most common malignancy observed was that of prostate, breast, colon and lung. In multivariate analysis they found that lung cancer was associated with 3-fold increase in mortality while in colon and prostate cancer mortality was not increased but had higher incidence of bleeding. Breast cancer patients' outcome was similar to those without cancer.

Epilogue

- The treatment of a severe or unstable heart condition in patients with simultaneous disease has priority because of its life-threatening nature
- Simultaneous surgical treatment of heart disease and cancer is often safe and feasible, but the effect of the use of ECC on cancer dissemination or on post-operative survival is still unclear
- If treatment by PCI is needed, the use of BMSs wherein DAPT is mandatory for 1 month and is preferred over DES which requires DAPT for at least 1 year. This causes a delay for cancer surgery, which is unacceptable from an oncologic

viewpoint. If coronary anatomy mandates use of DES CABG surgery (which does not need prolonged aggressive antiplatelet therapy) is a good option especially if underlying malignancy per se has good survival. Although the treatment of heart disease has priority because of its lifesaving aspect, the long-term postoperative survival in patients with simultaneous disease is largely determined by the stage of the tumor
- In patients with previously treated malignancy, the postoperative survival is determined by the time interval between the treatment of the tumor and heart surgery. With a longer time interval, the chance of cure of the cancer is higher
- Presence of lung cancer increases mortality three times after PCI
- Colon and prostate malignancy increase the risk of bleeding after PCI and hence need suitable adjustments in antiplatelet regimen
- Breast cancer patients undergoing PCI have similar outcomes as those without cancer.

REFERENCES

1. Iliescu C, Tsitlakidou D, Giza DE, et al. Primary Percutaneous Coronary Interventions in Cancer Patients. Cancer Research Frontiers. 2017;3(1):64-71.
2. Khakoo AY, Yeh ET. Therapy insight: Management of cardiovascular disease in patients with cancer and cardiac complications of cancer therapy. Nat Clin Pract Oncol. 2008;5(11):655-67.
3. Caine GJ, Stonelake PS, Lip GY, et al. The hypercoagulable state of malignancy: pathogenesis and current debate. Neoplasia. 2002;4(6):465-73.
4. Demers M, Krause DS, Schatzberg D, et al. Cancers predispose neutrophils to release extracellular DNA traps that contribute to cancer-associated thrombosis. Proc Natl Acad Sci U S A. 2012;109(32):13076-81.
5. Yeh ET, Bickford CL. Cardiovascular complications of cancer therapy: incidence, pathogenesis, diagnosis, and management. J Am Coll Cardiol. 2009;53(24):2231-47.
6. Tefferi A, Letendre L. Nilotinib treatment-associated peripheral artery disease and sudden death: yet another reason to stick to imatinib as front-line therapy for chronic myelogenous leukemia. Am J Hematol. 2011;86(7):610-1.
7. Burgdorf C, Nef HM, Haghi D, et al. Tako-tsubo (stress-induced) cardiomyopathy and cancer. Ann Intern Med. 2010;152(12):830-1.
8. Fajardo LF, Stewart JR. Coronary artery disease after radiation. N Engl J Med. 1972; 286(23):1265-6.
9. Yusuf SW, Daraban N, Abbasi N, et al. Treatment and outcomes of acute coronary syndrome in the cancer population. Clin Cardiol. 2012;35(7):443-50.
10. Patel B, Kloner RA, Ensley J, et al. 5-Fluorouracil cardiotoxicity: left ventricular dysfunction and effect of coronary vasodilators. Am J Med Sci. 1987;294(4):238-43.
11. Velders MA, Boden H, Hofma SH, et al. Outcome after ST elevation myocardial infarction in patients with cancer treated with primary percutaneous coronary intervention. Am J Cardiol. 2013;112:1867-72.
12. Landes U, Kornowski R, Bental T, et al. Long-term outcomes after percutaneous coronary interventions in cancer survivors. Coron Artery Dis. 2017;28(1):5-10.
13. Guddati AK, Joy PS, Kumar G. Analysis of outcomes of percutaneous coronary intervention in metastatic cancer patients with acute coronary syndrome over a 10-year period. J Cancer Res Clin Oncol. 2016;142(2):471-9.
14. Krone RJ. Managing coronary artery disease in the cancer patient. Prog Cardiovasc Dis. 2010;53(2):149-56.
15. Mauri L, Yeh RW, Kereiakes DJ. Duration of dual antiplatelet therapy after drug-eluting stents. N Engl J Med. 2015;372(14):1373-4.
16. Luzzatto G, Schafer AI. The prethrombotic state in cancer. Semin Oncol. 1990;17(2): 147-59.

17. Nathan S, Rao SV. Radial versus femoral access for percutaneous coronary intervention: implications for vascular complications and bleeding. Curr Cardiol Rep. 2012;14(4):502-9.
18. Lo TS, Ratib K, Chong AY, et al. Impact of access site selection and operator expertise on radiation exposure; a controlled prospective study. Am Heart J. 2012;164(4):455-61.
19. Iliescu C, Durand JB, Kroll M. Cardiovascular interventions in thrombocytopenic cancer patients. Tex Heart Inst J. 2011;38(3):259-60.
20. Yusuf SW, Iliescu C, Bathina JD, et al. Antiplatelet therapy and percutaneous coronary intervention in patients with acute coronary syndrome and thrombocytopenia. Tex Heart Inst J. 2010;37(3):336-40.
21. Mistiaen WP. Cancer in heart disease patients: what are the limitations in the treatment strategy? Future Cardiol. 2013;9(4):535-47.
22. Darwazah AK, Osman M, Sharabati B. Use of off-pump coronary artery bypass surgery among patients with malignant disease. J Card Surg. 2010;25(1):1-4.
23. Vieira RD, Pereira AC, Lima EG, et al. Cancer-related deaths among different treatment options in chronic coronary artery disease: results of a 6-year follow-up of the MASS II study. Coron Artery Dis. 2012;23:79-84.
24. Fu Q, Li QZ, Liang D, et al. Early and long-term results of combined cardiac surgery and neoplastic resection in patients with concomitant severe heart disease and neoplasms. Chinese Med J. 2011;124(13):1939-42.
25. La Francesca S, Frazier OH, Radovancevic B, et al. Concomitant cardiac and pulmonary operations for lung cancer. Tex Heart Inst J. 1995;22:296-300.
26. Tsuji Y, Morimoto N, Tanaka H, et al. Surgery for gastric cancer combined with cardiac and aortic surgery. Arch Surg. 2005;140:1109-14.
27. Özsoyler I, Yilik L, Bozok S, et al. Off-pump coronary artery bypass surgery in patients with coronary artery disease and malign neoplasia: results of ten patients and review of the literature. Heart Vessels. 2006;21;365-7.
28. Voltolini L, Rapicetta C, Luzzi L, et al. Lung resection for non-small cell lung cancer after prophylactic coronary angioplasty and stenting: short- and long-term results. Minerva Chir. 2012;67(1):77-85.
29. Shivaraju A, Patel V, Fonarow GC, et al. Temporal trends in gastrointestinal bleeding associated with percutaneous coronary intervention: analysis of the 1998–2006 Nationwide Inpatient Sample (NIS) database. Am Heart J. 2011;162:1062.e5-1068.e5.
30. Chan AO, Jim MH, Lam KF, et al. Prevalence of colorectal neoplasm among patients with newly diagnosed coronary artery disease. JAMA. 200;298:1412-9.
31. Neugut AI, Lebwohl B. Is the prevalence of colorectal neoplasm higher in patients with coronary artery disease? Nat Clin Pract Oncol. 2008;5:248-9.
32. Yang SY, Kim YS, Chung SJ, et al. Association between colorectal adenoma and coronary atherosclerosis detected by CT coronary angiography in Korean men; a cross-sectional study. J Gastroenterol Hepatol. 2010;25:1795-9.
33. Fleisher LA, Beckman JA, Brown KA, et al. ACC/AHA 2007 guidelines on perioperative cardiovascular evaluation and care for noncardiac surgery: executive summary. Circulation. 2007;116(17):1971-96.
34. Mishra PK, Pandey R, Shackcloth MJ, et al. Cardiac comorbidity is not a risk factor for mortality and morbidity following surgery for primary non-small cell lung cancer. Eur J Cardiothorac Surg. 2009;35(3):439-43.
35. Mistiaen W, Van Cauwelaert PH, Muylaert PH, et al. Effect of prior malignancy on survival after cardiac surgery. Ann Thorac Surg. 2004;77(5):1593-7.
36. Schoenmakers MC, van Boven WJ, van den Bosch J, et al. Comparison of on-pump or off-pump coronary artery revascularization with lung resection. Ann Thorac Surg. 2007;84:504-9.
37. Cathenis K, Hamerlijnck R, Vermassen F, et al. Concomitant cardiac surgery and pulmonary resection. Acta Chir Belg. 2009;109(3):306-11.
38. Zhang H, Wang D, Xiao F, et al. The impact of previous or concomitant myocardium revascularization on the outcomes of patients undergoing major non-cardiac surgery. Interact Cardiovasc Thorac Surg. 2009;9:788-92.
39. Voets AJ, Sheik Joesoef KS, Van Teeffelen ME. The influence of open-heart surgery on survival of patients with co-existent surgically amenable lung cancer (stage I and II). Eur Cardiothorac Surg. 1997;12:898-902.

40. Johnson JA, Landreneau RJ, Boley TM, et al. Should pulmonary lesions be resected at the time of open heart surgery? Am Surg. 1996;62(4):300-3.
41. Suzuki S, Usui A, Yoshida K, et al. Effect of cardiopulmonary bypass on cancer prognosis. Asian Cardiovasc Thorac Ann. 2010;18(6):536-40.
42. Nurözler F, Kutlu T, Kücük G. Off-pump coronary bypass for patients with concomitant malignancy. Circ J. 2006;70:1048-51.
43. Chan J, Rosenfeldt F, Chaudhuri K, et al. Cardiac surgery in patients with a history of malignancy: increased complication rate but similar mortality. Heart Lung Circ. 2012;21:255-9.
44. Samuels LE, Kaufman MS, Morris RJ, et al. Open heart surgery in patients with chronic lymphocytic leukemia. Leukemia Res. 1999;23:71-5.
45. Christiansen S, Schmid C, Loher A, et al. Impact of malignant hematological disorders on cardiac surgery. Cardiovasc Surg. 2000;8(2):149-52.
46. Fecher AM, Birdas TJ, Haybron D, et al. Cardiac operations in patients with hematologic malignancies. Eur J Cardiothorac Surg. 2004;25(4):537-40.
47. Yusuf SW, Sarfaraz A, Durand JB, et al. Management and outcomes of severe aortic stenosis in cancer patients. Am Heart J. 2011;161:1125-32.
48. Potapov EV, Zurbrügg HR, Herzke C, et al. Impact of cardiac surgery using cardiopulmonary bypass on course of chronic lymphatic leukemia: a case–control study. Ann Thorac Surg. 2002;74:384-9.
49. Hong RA, Limura T, Sumida KN, et al. Cardio-oncology/onco-cardiology. Clin Cardiol. 2010;33(12):733-7.
50. Schmitz KH, Prsonitz RG, Schwartz AL, et al. Prospective surveillance and management of cardiac toxicity and health in breast cancer survivors. Cancer. 2012;118(Suppl 8):2270-6.
51. Carrascal Y, Gualis J, Arévalo A, et al. [Cardiac surgery with extracorporeal circulation in cancer patients: influence on surgical morbidity and mortality and on survival]. Rev Esp Cardiol. 2008;61(4):369-75.
52. Yusuf WS, Razeghi P, Yeh ET. The diagnosis and management of cardiovascular disease in cancer patients. Curr Probl Cardiol. 2008;33:163-96.
53. Monsuez JJ, Charniot JC, Vignat N, et al. Cardiac side-effects of cancer chemotherapy. Int J Cardiol. 2010;144:3-15.
54. Hull MC, Morris CG, Pepine CJ, et al. Valvular dysfunction, and carotid, subclavian, and coronary artery disease in survivors of Hodgkin lymphoma. JAMA. 2003;290(21):2831-7.
55. Senkus-Konefka E, Jassem J. Cardiovascular effects of breast cancer radiotherapy. Cancer Treat Rev. 2007;33:578-93.
56. Wethal T, Lund MB, Edvardsen T, et al. Valvular dysfunction and left ventricular changes in Hodgkin's lymphoma survivors. A longitudinal study. Br J Cancer. 2009;101:575-81.
57. Handa N, McGregor CG, Danielson GK, et al. Coronary artery bypass grafting in patients with previous mediastinal radiation therapy. J Thorac Cardiovasc Surg. 1999;117:1136-43.
58. Hooning MJ, Botma A, Aleman BM, et al. Long-term risk of cardiovascular disease in 10-year survivors of breast cancer. J Natl Cancer Inst. 2007;99,365-75.
59. Chang AS, Smedira NG, Chang CL, et al. Cardiac surgery after mediastinal radiation: extent of exposure influences outcome. J Thorac Cardiovasc Surg. 2007;133:404-13.
60. Park CK, Xiaohong L, Starr J, et al. Cardiac morbidity and mortality in women with ductal carcinoma in situ of the breast treated with breast conservation therapy. Breast J. 2011;17(5):470-6.
61. Patt DA, Goodwin JS, Kup YF, et al. Cardiac morbidity of adjuvant radiotherapy for breast cancer. J Clin Oncol. 2005;23:7475-82.
62. McGale P, Darby SC, Hall P, et al. Incidence of heart disease in 35,000 women treated with radiotherapy for breast cancer in Denmark and Sweden. Radiother Oncol. 2011;100:167-75.
63. Cella L, Liuzzi R, Conson M, et al. Dosimetric predictors of asymptomatic heart valvular dysfunction following mediastinal irradiation for Hodgkin's lymphoma. Radiother Oncol. 2011;101:316-21.
64. Potts JE, Iliescu CA, Lopez Mattei JC, et al. PCI Outcomes in Cancer Patients, 2019. Available from: https://cardiomediquest.page.link/rqTHnwoo3KVWbvTu9

CHAPTER 9

Acute Coronary Syndrome with Connective Tissue Diseases

■ INTRODUCTION

Connective tissue diseases (CTDs) such as systemic lupus erythematosus (SLE), rheumatoid arthritis (RA) and systemic vasculitis are known to lead to premature coronary artery disease (CAD). In fact, accelerated CAD is a leading cause of mortality and morbidity in patients with CTD.[1] When compared to general population, younger patients with CTD and particularly SLE have a 50-fold risk of developing CAD.[2] Clinical atherosclerotic events and subclinical atherosclerosis have been most comprehensively studied in patients with SLE and RA.[3-5]

■ SYSTEMIC LUPUS ERYTHEMATOSUS AND CARDIOVASCULAR DISEASE

Even though long-term survival rates have considerably improved in patients with SLE, thanks to improved treatment regimens, mortality and morbidity continue to be high whenever these patients have a concurrent cardiovascular disease (CVD).[2] Manzi et al. reported that women with SLE have 5-6-fold heightened risk for CVD. They also reported that SLE patients in the age group of 35-44 years have a 50-fold increased risk for CVD.[2] A significant burden (more than 50%) of atherosclerosis has been reported in postmortem studies of patients of SLE, regardless of the cause of death.[1] Even though classic risk factors for CAD are associated with development of atherosclerosis in patients with SLE, two factors, namely, hypercholesterolemia and older age at diagnosis seem to have greater impact. Hypertension and diabetes that are more prevalent in SLE patients than in general population also lead to CAD in these patients.[2,6-8] In addition, smoking and longer duration of disease are also identified as risk factors for CAD in SLE patients.

A prospective cohort study by Esdaile et al. revealed that patients with SLE have a 7.5–17-fold risk for heart disease even after adjusting for baseline Framingham risk estimates.[9] It suggests that excess prevalence of traditional risk factors does not fully explain increased cardiovascular (CV) morbidity and mortality in patients with SLE. One other likely factor is therapy with steroids. Use of steroids in high dose can lead to many metabolic disorders such as central obesity, hypertension, glucose intolerance and alterations of lipid profiles. A study by Bulkeley et al. substantiates impact of steroid therapy on CAD in patients with SLE. In this study, use of steroids for more than a year was associated with increased incidence of atherosclerosis and CAD.[10] However, it has been noted that low-dose steroid (<10 mg daily) does not adversely affect the lipid profile in SLE patients. But, a steroid dose of >10 mg daily can cause increased levels of low-density lipoproteins (LDL) and triglycerides.[11] The effect of high-dose steroid on lipid profile was confirmed by two other studies.[12,13] Conversely, Okawa-Takatsuji et al. report that use of corticosteroids in SLE patients with renal dysfunction may result in lowered levels of lipoprotein.[14] This may benefit these patients because increased levels of lipoprotein are a known risk factor for developing heart disease.

In some patients with lupus, myocardial infarction (MI) may develop even before the diagnosis of SLE or shortly thereafter, suggesting that there may be a link between autoimmune inflammation and atherosclerosis. In the study by Urowitz et al. 31 of 1,848 patients had an MI. Of those, 23 patients had an MI either prior to SLE diagnosis or within the first 2 years of disease. This may be due to either delayed SLE diagnosis or actual accelerated CVD prior to SLE.[15]

A state of chronic inflammation in SLE due to mediators, cytokines, chemokines and adhesion molecules is considered another likely risk factor contributing to atherosclerosis and eventually heart disease.[16-18] Moreover, the autoimmune nature of the disease process in SLE is characterized by production of various autoantibodies that are associated with risk for thrombosis (Flowchart 1).[19]

PREVENTION AND TREATMENT

Lifestyle Modifications

Prevention of CAD in patients with SLE would include avoiding modifiable risk factors by encouraging them to make modifications in lifestyle. These patients must be advised to avoid smoking cigarettes, to exercise regularly, and to achieve a body mass index of <25 kg/m² and to follow dietary measures to improve lipid profiles.

Statins

In view of their pleiotropic effects including anti-inflammatory, antithrombotic and plaque-stabilizing activities, statins are considered ideal for

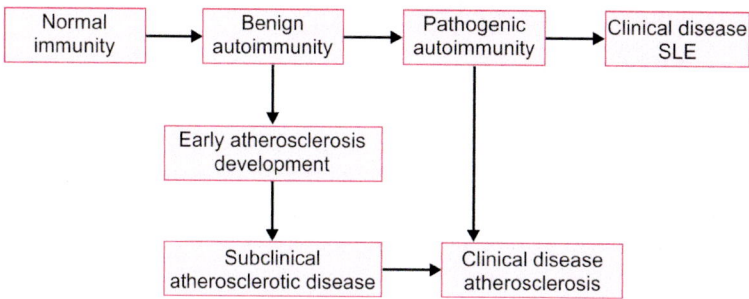

(SLE: systemic lupus erythematosus)

FLOWCHART 1: Possible pathophysiology of CAD in SLE.

lowering lipids in patients with SLE. Atorvastatin and fluvastatin are preferred in patients with SLE and renal impairment because these do not require dosage adjustment even when there is significant reduction in glomerular filtration rate (GFR).

Hydroxychloroquine

Even though the impact of hydroxychloroquine on reducing CAD risk in SLE patients is not conclusively demonstrated, several lines of evidence suggest that it may have some beneficial effect.

Control of Hypertension

Hypertension is an important risk factor for heart disease in patients with SLE and hence aggressive treatment is recommended. The goal blood pressure (BP) in SLE patients is the same as in those without it. It is especially true when a patient with SLE has diabetes or chronic renal dysfunction. The choice of antihypertensive agent in some parts depends on coexisting illness. Nifedipine is recommended for patients with Raynaud's phenomenon, while ACE inhibitors are suggested in patients with chronic kidney disease.

Prophylactic Use of Aspirin

As in patients without SLE, use of low-dose aspirin for prophylaxis in patients with SLE is individualized and depends on estimated risk of a first CV event.

Minimizing Glucocorticoid Dose

Since glucocorticoids are known to contribute toward CAD risk factors by worsening hypertension, hyperlipidemia and diabetes, their dosage must be reduced as soon as possible.

RHEUMATOID ARTHRITIS AND CARDIAC DISEASE

Rheumatoid arthritis is the most common inflammatory rheumatic disease with a worldwide prevalence of 0.5–2%. This crippling disease has a reduced life expectancy with a standardized mortality ratio of 2.0.[1] Premature atherosclerosis accounts for 40–50% of the deaths in patient of RA.[20,21] A recent meta-analysis by Levy et al. demonstrated that patients with RA have a 1.63-fold increased risk of myocardial ischemia compared to the general population.[22] The predisposition of RA patients to CV risk is multifactorial in nature. Chronic inflammation in RA leads to derangement of lipids as in SLE. It has been demonstrated that patients of RA who test positive for rheumatoid factor have a 50% higher CV mortality when compared to age- and sex-matched controls.[21] In addition, a higher baseline C-reactive protein levels predict increased CV mortality—suggesting that inflammation plays an important role in the pathogenesis of CVD.[23] It is demonstrated that atherosclerosis in RA patients correlates with total duration of the disease—indicating that prolonged exposure to chronic inflammation predisposes to CAD.[24] It is also suggested, interestingly, that the risk of CAD may precede the onset of RA[25] and that it is probably related to low-grade inflammation before clinical synovitis sets in. Del Rincon et al. noted in their study that systemic inflammation is the key risk factor in RA patients less than 54 years.[24] Krishnan et al. and Choi et al. noted in their study that methotrexate therapy, which is the mainstay of treatment in RA, reduced the cardiovascular mortality by as much as 70%.[26,27] Similarly, antitumor necrosis factor agents apparently reduce the risk of CAD.[28] All of these studies seem to suggest that adequate control of inflammation in RA may be an important mechanism to diminish risk of CAD.

However, the development of accelerated atherosclerosis is less obvious in patients of systemic sclerosis. Also, there is little evidence for macrovascular complications such as stroke and MI in systemic sclerosis.

Warrington et al. in their study observed that RA patients were at increased risk of multivessel CAD and had trend toward increased mortality, though rate of CV events was similar (Figs. 1A and B).[29]

CORONARY ARTERY DISEASE IN RHEUMATOID ARTHRITIS: IMPLICATIONS FOR PREVENTION AND MANAGEMENT

The following are some of the issues that are of particular concern in RA that may affect CV risk:
- Effects of systemic inflammation on CAD
- Issues related to concomitant use of low-dose aspirin with nonsteroidal anti-inflammatory drugs (NSAIDs) or cyclooxygenase (COX)-2 selective inhibitors

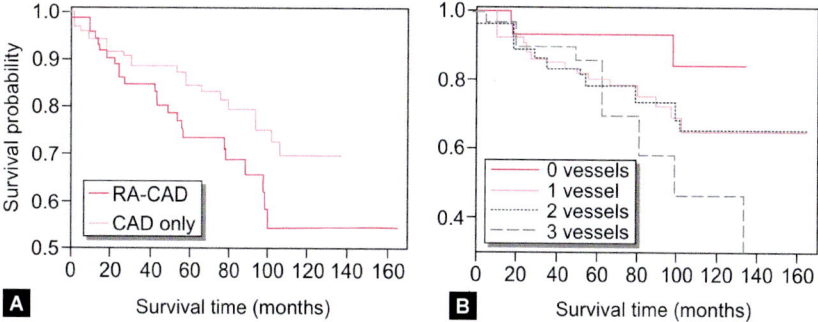

FIGS. 1A AND B: Decrease in survival in patients of RA who have CAD and survival further decreases with increase in CAD severity.

Source: Warrington KJ, Kent PD, Frye RL, et al. Rheumatoid arthritis is an independent risk factor for multi-vessel coronary artery disease: a case control study. Arthritis Res Ther. 2005;7(5):R984-R991.

- Benefits and adverse effects of glucocorticoids and other anti-RA therapies. Various RA therapies include nonbiologic as well as biologic disease-modifying antirheumatic drugs (DMARDs).

Control of Blood Pressure

Glucocorticoids, leflunomide, and NSAIDs used in RA therapy are prone to modestly increase BP.[30-32] Hence, close monitoring of BP before and after initiation of such therapies combined with judicious adjustment of dosage to maintain optimal BP is recommended to reduce risk of CAD. Early initiation of DMARDs may help to avoid regular use of NSAIDs and glucocorticoids.

Exercise

It may be difficult or even impossible for the patients of RA with active synovitis to perform desired levels of aerobic exercise.

Lipid-lowering with Statins

Primary and secondary prevention of CVD with statin therapy is recommended in patients with RA using the same guidelines as for those without RA.

Low-dose Aspirin

Use of low-dose aspirin for prevention of CVD in RA patients does not differ from those without RA in general population. However, it affects the use of NSAIDs.

In patients of RA, use of low-dose aspirin for primary and secondary prevention of CVD may be complicated by the following issues:
- Nonselective and nonaspirin NSAIDs may interfere with beneficial effects of low-dose aspirin

- The COX-2 selective NSAIDs do not seem to interfere with the antiplatelet effect of aspirin. Moreover, risk of coronary incidents is apparently less with celecoxib than with rofecoxib. Nonetheless, it is recommended to avoid use of COX-2 selective drugs in patients without proven CAD until the issue of their CV safety is settled
- When low-dose aspirin is combined with COX-2 selective agents, the incidence of hemorrhage in the gastrointestinal (GI) tract is similar to the patients treated with nonselective NSAIDs. It is not certain whether low-dose aspirin brings down CV risk in patients who are treated with COX-2 selective agent.

IMPLICATIONS FOR RA THERAPEUTIC DRUG SELECTION

In patients of CAD receiving warfarin or other vitamin K antagonists, use of nonselective NSAID is associated with increased risk of bleeding from GI tract. In such a context, celecoxib, which does not interfere with platelet aggregation, is recommended in lowest effective dose. Use of lowest effective dose of glucocorticoids instead of a COX-2 selective NSAID is another alternative suggested to avoid risk of GI bleed. A similar approach is recommended for those patients who are on dual anti-platelet therapy with aspirin and a $P2Y_{12}$ inhibitor such as clopidogrel, prasugrel, or ticagrelor.

NSAIDs and Cardiovascular Events

The use of NSAIDs is associated with an increased risk of CVD events in patients with and without CVD. The increase in absolute risk is higher in those with established CVD due to the higher baseline risk.

The magnitude of the increase in relative and absolute risks is best illustrated by a 2013 meta-analysis of predominantly individual participant data from randomized trials that compared nonselective NSAIDs or selective COX-2 inhibitors (coxibs) with either placebo or another non-selective NSAID or coxib.[33] The analysis [Coxib and traditional NSAID Trialists' (CNT) Collaboration] utilized data from over 300,000 individuals in over 600 trials. In these trials, only 9% had a history of CVD. After follow-up of approximately 1 year, the meta-analysis found:
- Major CV events (a composite of nonfatal MI, nonfatal stroke, or vascular death) were increased compared with placebo for high-dose diclofenac and for the coxibs largely due to increase in major coronary heart disease events. A similar but statistically nonsignificant increase in risk was observed with high-dose ibuprofen compared with placebo. The use of high-dose naproxen did not result in an increase in major CV events. There was a trend toward an increase in vascular death, as an individual endpoint, with diclofenac, the coxibs and ibuprofen compared with

placebo. Risk of vascular death was not significantly increased by use of naproxen compared with placebo
- The study data permitted estimates of the excess absolute risk of a major vascular event or death associated with use of these agents. For patients at low-CV risk (baseline risk of 0.5% per year), the use of diclofenac, ibuprofen, or a coxib resulted in an excess of two events per 1,000 persons per year; naproxen was not associated with any excess risk. This small increase in risk will rarely influence the decision whether to use one of these drugs for short-term analgesia.

Drug Comparisons

For any given patient, the baseline risks for CV events and GI bleeding need to be considered prior to recommending a specific agent. Available evidence suggests that high-dose naproxen may have the best CV risk profile among all NSAIDs and that celecoxib may have the best profile with regard to GI risk.[34]

NSAID in Rheumatoid Arthritis

The impact of nonselective NSAID on CV outcomes in RA patients has not yet been studied extensively. However, limited available data suggests that CVD risk of NSAID is probably less in RA patients when compared to general population. Nonselective NSAIDs have no significant CV risk benefit in general population. On the contrary, available data suggests that diclofenac and probably other agents have an adverse effect on CVD outcomes. COX-2 selective NSAIDs are associated with heightened risk for CVD.

LIMITED GLUCOCORTICOID EXPOSURE

When long-term treatment with glucocorticoids is necessitated, it is desirable to taper the dose as quickly as possible. Lowest effective dose of 5–10 mg/day of prednisone or its equivalent is recommended based on disease activity. Supraphysiologic dose of glucocorticoids is associated with increased rate of myocardial ischemia, heart failure, stroke and all-cause mortality. These effects are mediated at least in parts by increasing the lipoprotein levels. Such ill effects of chronic glucocorticoid therapy are typically seen at doses of 7.5 mg/day or higher. But the adverse effects are reported even at a lower dose.

TREATMENT OF ANGINA AND ACUTE CORONARY SYNDROME

The medical management of patients with RA along with angina and/or acute coronary syndrome does not vary much from such management in patients without RA. However, patients of RA who present with acute coronary syndrome may have poorer outcome than the general population.

■ REVASCULARIZATION IN PATIENTS WITH RA

Indications for PCI or CABG in patients with RA are same as in patients without RA. However, long-term outcomes are poorer in patients with RA because of target vessel failure leading to frequent need for reintervention. This could be explained by chronic inflammation, which is the hallmark of RA.

■ PRIMARY SYSTEMIC VASCULITIS AND RISK FOR CVD

Primary systemic vasculitis (PSV) comprises a range of conditions characterized by immune-mediated, necrotizing inflammation of the vessel wall leading to stenosis, and occlusion of vessels of different size. This leads to ischemic complications in various organs. The necrotizing inflammation of the vessel wall may also lead to aneurysmal dilatation and rupture of the vessels resulting in hemorrhagic complications. Depending on the size of the vessel involved, PSV can be classified into small, medium, or large-vessel vasculitis. A few available reports regarding CV events related to vasculitis pertain to Kawasaki disease (KD) and Henoch–Schonlein purpura. A study by Dhillon et al. reported reduction in flow-mediated dilatation (FMD) and endothelium-dependent response in KD compared to healthy controls. Proatherogenic lipid profile (low HDL and high LDL) was also reported in these patients.[35] Accelerated atherosclerosis of the carotid arteries similar to SLE is reported in patients with Takayasu's arteritis.[36] This incidence is greater than healthy controls. Systemic inflammation with sustained release of inflammatory cytokines and adhesion molecules favors development of atherosclerosis.

■ PRIMARY ANTIPHOSPHOLIPID SYNDROME

Primary antiphospholipid syndrome (PAPS) is a prothrombotic condition. It is characterized by recurrent thrombosis of the arteries and veins and morbidity in pregnancy. Laboratory tests reveal persistently elevated antiphospholipid antibodies. Even though PAPS is primarily a thrombotic condition, accelerated atherosclerosis is not explained by conventional risk factors. It may be due to the presence of autoantibodies such as anti-oxLDL and anti-$β2$ glycoprotein-I ($β2$GPI).[37]

■ SJÖGREN'S SYNDROME AND CARDIOVASCULAR RISK

Sjögren's syndrome is an autoimmune disease. It is characterized by production of autoantibodies and cellular infiltration of the exocrine glands. Primary involvement of CV system is rare in Sjögren's syndrome unlike other CTD. There is no formal study confirming or refuting increased CVD risk in this condition.

ADULT INFLAMMATORY MYOSITIS

Polymyositis and dermatomyositis are immune-mediated conditions affecting primarily the skeletal muscle. These usually require a high dose of corticosteroids for a prolonged period. In addition, inflammatory myocarditis is a recognized entity associated with inflammatory myositis.[38] However, there are no significant epidemiological studies regarding association between these conditions and CVD.

Epilogue

- Connective tissue diseases especially SLE and RA have increased prevalence of CVD. This can be partially due deranged risk factor profile due to steroids but mainly due to underlying chronic inflammation
- Disease-modifying agents in RA can reduce the risk of CAD
- Most NSAIDs including COX-2 inhibitors increase the risk of CVD. Naproxen has best CV safety, while celecoxib has the best GI safety
- Steroids should be prescribed in the lowest possible dose.

REFERENCES

1. Al Husain A, Bruce IN. Risk factors for coronary heart disease in connective tissue diseases. Ther Adv Musculoskel Dis. 2010;2(3):145-53.
2. Manzi S, Meilahn EN, Rairie JE, et al. Age-specific incidence rates of myocardial infarction and angina in women with systemic lupus erythematosus: Comparison with the Framingham study. Am J Epidemiol. 1997;145(5):408-15.
3. Haque SA, Mirjafari HA, Bruce IN. Atherosclerosis in rheumatoid arthritis and systemic lupus erythematosus. Curr Opin Lipidol. 2008;19(4):338-43.
4. El-Magadmi M, Bodill H, Ahmad Y, et al. Systemic lupus erythematosus: An independent risk factor for endothelial dysfunction in women. Circulation. 2004;110(4):399-404.
5. Roman MJ, Shanker BA, Davis A, et al. Prevalence and correlates of accelerated atherosclerosis in systemic lupus erythematosus. New Engl J Med. 2003;349(25):2399-406.
6. Svenungsson E, Jensen-Urstad K, Heimbürger M, et al. Risk factors for cardiovascular disease in systemic lupus erythematosus. Circulation. 2001;104:1887-93.
7. Gladman DD, Urowitz MB. Morbidity in systemic lupus erythematosus. J Rheumatol. 1987;14(Suppl 13):223-6.
8. Bruce IN, Urowitz MB, Gladman DD, et al. Risk factors for coronary heart disease in women with systemic lupus erythematosus: The Toronto risk factor study. Arthritis Rheum. 2003;48:3159-67.
9. Esdaile JM, Abrahamowicz M, Grodzicky T, et al. Traditional Framingham risk factors fail to fully account for accelerated atherosclerosis in systemic lupus erythematosus. Arthritis Rheum. 2001;44:2331-7.
10. Bulkeley BH, Roberts WC. The heart in systemic lupus erythematosus and the changes induced in it by corticosteroid therapy. A study of 36 necropsy patients. Am J Med Sci. 1975;58(2):243-64.
11. MacGregor AJ, Dhillon VB, Binder A, et al. Fasting lipids and anticardiolipin antibodies as risk factors for vascular disease in systemic lupus erythematosus. Ann Rheum Dis. 1992;51:152-5.
12. Bruce IN, Urowitz MB, Gladman DD, et al. Natural history of hypercholesterolemia in systemic lupus erythematosus. J Rheumatol. 1999;26:2137-43.

13. Keng Hong L, Ee Tzun K, Pao Hsii F, et al. Lipid profiles in patients with systemic lupus erythematosus. J Rheumatol. 1994;21:1264-7.
14. Okawa-Takatsuji M, Aotsuka S, Sumiya M, et al. Clinical significance of the serum lipoprotein(a) level in patients with systemic lupus erythematosus: Its elevation during disease flare. Clin Exp Rheumatol. 1996;14:531-6.
15. Urowitz MB, Gladman DD, Anderson NM, et al. Cardiovascular events prior to or early after diagnosis of systemic lupus erythematosus in the systemic lupus international collaborating clinics cohort. Lupus Sci Med. 2016;3(1):e000143.
16. Pearson TA, Mensah GA, Alexander RW, et al. Markers of inflammation and cardiovascular disease: Application to clinical and public health practice: A statement for healthcare professionals from the Centers for Disease Control and Prevention and the American Heart Association. Circulation. 2003;107:499-511.
17. Ridker PM, Hennekens CH, Buring JE, et al. C-reactive protein and other markers of inflammation in the prediction of cardiovascular disease in women. New Engl J Med. 2000;342:836-43.
18. Hansson GK. Immune mechanisms in atherosclerosis. Arteriosclerosis Thromb Vasc Biol. 2001;21:1876-90.
19. Frostegard J. Atherosclerosis in patients with autoimmune disorders. Arterioscler Thromb Vasc Biol. 2005;25:1776-85.
20. Sihvonen S, Korpela M, Laippala P, et al. Death rates and causes of death in patients with rheumatoid arthritis: A population-based study. Scand J Rheumatol. 2004;33:221-7.
21. Wallberg-Jonsson S, Ohman ML, Dahlqvist SR. Cardiovascular morbidity and mortality in patients with seropositive rheumatoid arthritis in northern Sweden. J Rheumatol. 1997;24:445-51.
22. Levy L, Fautrel B, Barnetche T, et al. Incidence and risk of fatal myocardial infarction and stroke events in rheumatoid arthritis patients. A systematic review of the literature. Clin Exp Rheumatol. 2008;26:673-9.
23. Goodson NJ, Symmons DPM, Scott DGI, et al. Baseline levels of C-reactive protein and prediction of death from cardiovascular disease in patients with inflammatory polyarthritis: A ten-year follow-up study of a primary care-based inception cohort. Arthritis Rheum. 2005;52:2293-9.
24. Del Rincon I, Williams K, Stern MP, et al. High incidence of cardiovascular events in a rheumatoid arthritis cohort not explained by traditional cardiac risk factors. Arthritis Rheum. 2001;44:2737-45.
25. Maradit-Kremers H, Cynthia SC, Paulo JN, et al. Increased unrecognized coronary heart disease and sudden deaths in rheumatoid arthritis: A population-based cohort study. Arthritis Rheum. 2005;52:402-11.
26. Krishnan E, Lingala VB, Singh G. Declines in mortality from acute myocardial infarction in successive incidence and birth cohorts of patients with rheumatoid arthritis. Circulation. 2004;110:1774-9.
27. Choi HK, Hernan MA, Seeger JD, et al. Methotrexate and mortality in patients with rheumatoid arthritis: A prospective study. Lancet. 2002;359:1173-7.
28. Dixon WG, Watson KD, Lunt M, et al. Reduction in the incidence of myocardial infarction in patients with rheumatoid arthritis who respond to anti-tumor necrosis factor alpha therapy: Results from the British Society for Rheumatology Biologics Register. Arthritis Rheum. 2007;56:2905-12.
29. Warrington KJ, Kent PD, Frye RL, et al. Rheumatoid arthritis is an independent risk factor for multi-vessel coronary artery disease: A case control study. Arthritis Res Ther. 2005;7(5):R984-91.
30. Liao KP, Malhotra R. UPTODATE march 2018.
31. Smolen JS, Kalden JR, Scott DL, et al. Efficacy and safety of leflunomide compared with placebo and sulphasalazine in active rheumatoid arthritis: a double-blind, randomised, multicentre trial. European Leflunomide Study Group. Lancet. 1999;353:259.

32. Strand V, Cohen S, Schiff M, et al. Treatment of active rheumatoid arthritis with leflunomide compared with placebo and methotrexate. Leflunomide Rheumatoid Arthritis Investigators Group. Arch Intern Med. 1999;159:2542.
33. Bhala N, Emberson J, Merhi A, et al. Vascular and upper gastrointestinal effects of non-steroidal anti-inflammatory drugs: meta-analyses of individual participant data from randomised trials. Lancet. 2013;382:769.
34. Chan FKL, Ching JYL, Tse YK, et al. Gastrointestinal safety of celecoxib versus naproxen in patients with cardiothrombotic diseases and arthritis after upper gastrointestinal bleeding (CONCERN): an industry-independent, double-blind, double-dummy, randomised trial. Lancet. 2017;389:2375.
35. Cheung YF, Yung TC, Tam SCF, et al. Novel and traditional cardiovascular risk factors in children after Kawasaki disease: Implications for premature atherosclerosis. J Am Coll Cardiol. 2004;43:120-4.
36. Seyahi E, Ugurlu S, Cumali R, et al. Atherosclerosis in Takayasu arteritis. Ann Rheum Dis. 2006;65:1202-7.
37. Belizna CC, Richard V, Primard E, et al. Early atheroma in primary and secondary antiphospholipid syndrome: An intrinsic finding. Semin Arthritis Rheum. 2008;37:373-80.
38. White PG, Podgorski MR, Mcleod TIF, et al. Acute myocarditis causing fatal ventricular arrhythmia in treated polymyositis. Rheumatology. 1988;27:399-402.

10
CHAPTER

Acute Coronary Syndrome with Human Immunodeficiency Virus Infections

INTRODUCTION

Rapid developments in the recent times in the treatment of human deficiency virus (HIV) infections have significantly improved the survival rates. The patients afflicted with HIV were at an increased risk of premature death from opportunistic infections and cardiac disease including heart failure before the combined combination antiretroviral therapy (cART) was introduced into the treatment arsenal. With the advent of cART, the prognosis of retroviral infection has dramatically altered. Presently, life-expectancy in HIV-infected patients is almost the same as general population. However, these patients now face high rate of cardiac complications including heart failure. A higher calculated risk of cardiovascular disease (CVD) is now reported among survivors of retroviral disease when compared to age-matched, HIV-negative population.[1] The higher CVD risk in this group is due to following reasons:
- Atherogenic lipid profile
- Insulin resistance from chronic cART
- Higher incidence of traditional risk factors of CVD such as cigarette smoking, dyslipidemia and diabetes

In addition, the infection with HIV is itself a risk factor for coronary artery disease (CAD) due to the chronic inflammatory milieu.[2] Elevated inflammatory markers are reported even in patients receiving antiretroviral therapy.[3]

EPIDEMIOLOGY

A recent meta-analysis examining the risk of CVD in patients with HIV without treatment found that the risk of CVD was 61% higher in comparison to the general population—not infected by HIV.[4]

ETIOLOGY OF INCREASED CARDIOVASCULAR DISEASE RISK

Complex pathophysiological mechanisms are involved in increased risk of ischemic heart disease in patients infected with HIV. The mechanisms are likely to be a combination of traditional as well as novel risk factors.

Antiretroviral Therapy

There is a well-established association between cART and cardiovascular risk.[5-9] Following are the three principal classes of antiretroviral therapy:
1. Protease inhibitors (PIs)
2. Nucleoside reverse transcriptase inhibitors (NRTIs)
3. Non-nucleoside reverse transcriptase inhibitors (NNRTIs)

The Data Collection on Adverse Events of Anti-HIV Drugs (DAD) study[6] revealed that there was an incremental increase in the incidence of MI with increasing exposure of combination antiretroviral therapy—especially the PIs.[7] After 6 years of exposure to PIs, the incidence of MI increased from 1.5 to 6 events per 1,000 person years in patients infected with HIV. It was with an adjusted relative risk of 1.16 for every year of exposure to the PIs.[7] In addition, recent use of NRTIs such as abacavir and didanosine have been shown to increase the risk of MI by 90% and 49% respectively. This is in comparison to those patients who have never used these drugs or stopped taking them more than 6 months before.[9] The largest meta-analysis so far in this connection consisted of 26 randomized control trials and a total of 9,868 subjects. This meta-analysis could not find any connection between abacavir cause and risk of MI.[10] Similarly, no association between exposure to NNRTIs and increased risk of MI has been reported.[6,8] However, cumulative exposure to indinavir or lopinavir-ritonavir has been shown to be associated with an increased risk of MI. Certain not so frequently prescribed antiviral agents such as nelfinavir or saquinavir are not associated with any heightened risk of MI.

However, there is a paradox here. Continuous exposure to cART is associated with reduced risk of myocardial infarction. It was observed that the subjects participating in the DAD study who received cART had a 2% risk of myocardial infarction at 3 year.[11] A less than 1.5% reduction was observed in the 3-year risk of MI when these subjects stopped cART. In contrast, there is a 3-year risk of AIDS or death of 5–10% in people receiving cART; a rate of 25–35% in people not receiving cART and 22–29% in people receiving cART but who ceased treatment midway.[11] The SMART trial (Strategies for Management of Antiretroviral Therapy) reported that cessation of ART lead to a paradoxical higher risk of myocardial infarction.

Human Immunodeficiency Virus and Risk of Coronary Artery Disease

Human immunodeficiency virus infection is thought to precipitate a pro-atherogenic state through the interplay of multiple mechanisms.[12] The untreated HIV infection is characterized by chronic immune activation and inflammation. As a result, CRP and IL6 levels are elevated—leading to higher incidence of CAD.[13,14] In addition, higher levels of D-dimer, fibrinogen and other coagulation markers leading to a procoagulant state is thought to contribute toward increased risk of CVD in patients with HIV.[12]

Dyslipidemia

Infection with HIV is known to cause a decrease in cardioprotective high-density lipoproteins (HDLs).[15,16] The reduced levels of HDL results in a modest state of dyslipidemia. It is independent of ART. However, most of the dyslipidemic state results from cART.[17] Compared to PIs and NNRTIs, the changes in lipid levels caused by NRTIs are mild. Etravirine which is a newer NNRTI, has little effect on the patient's lipid profile.[18]

Insulin Resistance/Metabolic Syndrome

A high prevalence of glucose metabolism is reported in patients infected with HIV. As much as 25–30% of the patients infected with HIV have insulin resistance. Incidence of diabetes among this population is reported to be 2–8%.[19-21] HIV infection by itself does not significantly increase the risk of diabetes.[22] However, a significant association is reported between cART and abnormal glucose metabolism. The abnormalities in glucose metabolism are known to increase with cumulative exposure to cART.[23]

Blood Pressure

As much as one-third of the patients infected with HIV suffer from hypertension. It is associated with insulin resistance and metabolic syndrome.[16] However, there is a controversy regarding incidence of hypertension in HIV patients when compared to those without HIV infection.[24]

Cessation of Cigarette Smoking

Compared to general population, the prevalence of cigarette smoking is 2–3 times higher in HIV-infected patients.[25,26] Moreover, the impact of smoking on the risk of MI in HIV is greater than the other traditional risk factors for CVD.[7,27]

Lipid-lowering Therapy

Since there is a significant risk of harmful interactions, simvastatin and lovastatin should not be prescribed along with PIs.[28] Similarly, caution must be exercised while prescribing atorvastatin in combination with protease inhibitors—lowest possible dose should be used.[28] Even though rosuvastatin is not metabolized by the CYP3A4 enzyme, it should be used with caution and at a low dose when a concomitant use of PIs is required. Rosuvastatin is proven to be more effective in lowering LDL-C and triglycerides (TG) than pravastatin in patients with HIV infection. Moreover, it does not cause any severe adverse effects.[29]

Management of Coronary Artery Disease

Majority of the patients with HIV are treated with conventional methods. These are:[30]
- Percutaneous coronary intervention (PCI, 25-76%)
- Coronary artery bypass grafting (CABG, 4-18%)
- Medical therapy alone (10-20%).

There is no significant difference in major adverse cardiac and cerebrovascular events (MACCEs) and clinical restenosis at 1-year follow-up between the HIV and non-HIV subjects undergoing treatment for acute coronary syndrome (ACS). However, recurrent ACS and primary PCI is more frequent in patients infected with HIV.[31] However, when the follow-up period is extended to 2 years after pooling the results of multiple studies, the incidence of acute MI in patients with previous ACS is almost 10%.[32,33] Whenever a HIV-infected patient is subjected to PCI, drug-eluting stents (DESs) should be implanted in order to reduce major adverse cardiac events (MACEs).[34,35] Conventional therapy with dual antiplatelet therapy must follow for a period of 6-12 months after target-vessel and target-lesion revascularization. Clopidogrel is activated by the CYP2C19 enzyme system which is inhibited by the NNRTI—etravirine. Hence, combination of etravirine and clopidogrel is discouraged even though a formal assessment of the interaction between them is not done so far.[35] The treating physicians should be aware of the potential interactions between the newer antiplatelet agents such as prasugrel[36] or ticagrelor[37] and ritonavir. This caution should be exercised despite the recent moves to use more potent antiplatelet agents in the general population after a stent implantation.

Epilogue
- Prevalence of CAD is more in retroviral-infected patients due to multiple factors
- Some antiretroviral medicines too contribute to increased CAD risk
- Treatment of ACS in these patients is similar to that of general population
- Recurrence of coronary events is higher in these patients despite optimal treatment
- Combination of clopidogrel with etravirine, prasugrel or ticagrelor with ritonavir needs to be discouraged.

■ REFERENCES

1. Kaplan RC, Kingsley LA, Sharrett AR, et al. Ten-year predicted coronary heart disease risk in HIV-infected men and women. Clin Infect Dis. 2007;45:1074-81.
2. Currier JS, Taylor A, Boyd F, et al. Coronary heart disease in HIV-infected individuals. J Acquir Immune Defic Syndr. 2003;33:506-12.
3. Freiberg MS, Chang CC, Kuller LH, et al. HIV infection and the risk of acute myocardial infarction. JAMA Intern Med. 2013;173:614-22.
4. Islam FM, Wu J, Jansson J, et al. Relative risk of cardiovascular disease among people living with HIV: a systematic review and meta-analysis. HIV Med. 2012;13: 453-68.
5. Lang S, Mary-Krause M, Simon A, et al. HIV replication and immune status are independent predictors of the risk of myocardial infarction in HIV-infected individuals. Clin Infect Dis. 2012;55:600-7.
6. Friis-Møller N, Sabin CA, Weber R, et al. Combination antiretroviral therapy and the risk of myocardial infarction. N Engl J Med. 2003;349:1993-2003.
7. Friis-Møller N, Reiss P, Sabin CA, et al. Class of antiretroviral drugs and the risk of myocardial infarction. N Engl J Med. 2007;356:1723-35.
8. Worm SW, Sabin C, Weber R, et al. Risk of myocardial infarction in patients with HIV infection exposed to specific individual antiretroviral drugs from the 3 major drug classes: the data collection on adverse events of anti-HIV drugs (D:A:D) study. J Infect Dis. 2010;201:318-30.
9. Sabin CA, Worm SW, Weber R, et al. Use of nucleoside reverse transcriptase inhibitors and risk of myocardial infarction in HIV-infected patients enrolled in the D:A:D study: a multi-cohort collaboration. Lancet. 2008;371:1417-26.
10. Ding X, Andraca-Carrera E, Cooper C, et al. No association of abacavir use with myocardial infarction: findings of an FDA meta-analysis. J Acquir Immune Defic Syndr. 2012;61:441-7.
11. Law M, Friis-Møller N, Weber R, et al. Modelling the 3-year risk of myocardial infarction among participants in the Data Collection on Adverse Events of Anti-HIV Drugs (DAD) study. HIV Med. 2003;4:1-10.
12. Baker JV, Lundgren JD. Cardiovascular implications from untreated human immuno-deficiency virus infection. Eur Heart J. 2011;32:945-51.
13. Triant VA, Meigs JB, Grinspoon SK. Association of C-reactive protein and HIV infection with acute myocardial infarction. J Acquir Immune Defic Syndr. 2009;51:268-73.
14. Kuller LH, Tracy R, Belloso W, et al. Inflammatory and coagulation biomarkers and mortality in patients with HIV infection. PLoS Med. 2008;5:e203.
15. Duprez DA, Kuller LH, Tracy R, et al. Lipoprotein particle subclasses, cardiovascular disease and HIV infection. Atherosclerosis. 2009;207:524-9.
16. Gazzaruso C, Bruno R, Garzaniti A, et al. Hypertension among HIV patients: prevalence and relationships to insulin resistance and metabolic syndrome. J Hypertens. 2003;21: 1377-82.
17. Badiou S, Merle De Boever C, Dupuy AM, et al. Decrease in LDL size in HIV-positive adults before and after lopinavir/ritonavir containing regimen: an index of atherogenicity? Atherosclerosis. 2003;168:107-13.
18. Girard PM, Campbell TB, Grinsztejn B, et al. Pooled week 96 results of the phase III DUET-1 and DUET-2 trials of etravirine: further analysis of adverse events and laboratory abnormalities of special interest. HIV Med. 2012;13:427-35.
19. Brown TT, Cole SR, Li X, et al. Antiretroviral therapy and the prevalence and incidence of diabetes mellitus in the multicenter AIDS cohort study. Arch Intern Med. 2005;165: 1179-84.

20. Wand H, Calmy A, Carey DL, et al. Metabolic syndrome, cardiovascular disease and type 2 diabetes mellitus after initiation of antiretroviral therapy in HIV infection. AIDS. 2007;21:2445-53.
21. Justman JE, Benning L, Danoff A, et al. Protease inhibitor use and the incidence of diabetes mellitus in a large cohort of HIV infected women. J Acquir Immune Defic Syndr. 2003;32:298-302.
22. Butt AA, McGinnis K, Rodriguez-Barradas MC, et al. HIV infection and the risk of diabetes mellitus. AIDS. 2009;23:1227-34.
23. De Wit S, Sabin CA, Weber R, et al. Incidence and risk factors for new-onset diabetes in HIV-infected patients: the Data Collection on Adverse Events of Anti-HIV Drugs (D:A:D) study. Diabetes Care. 2008;31:1224-9.
24. Jericó C, Knobel H, Montero M, et al. Hypertension in HIV-infected patients: prevalence and related factors. Am J Hypertens. 2005;18:1396-1401.
25. Helleberg M, Afzal S, Kronborg G, et al. Mortality attributable to smoking among HIV-1-infected individuals: a nationwide, population-based cohort study. Clin Infect Dis. 2013;56:727-34.
26. Tesoriero JM, Gieryic SM, Carrascal A, et al. Smoking among HIV positive New Yorkers: prevalence, frequency, and opportunities for cessation. AIDS Behav. 2010;14:824-35.
27. Lifson AR, Neuhaus J, Arribas JR, et al. Smoking-related health risks among persons with HIV in the Strategies for Management of Antiretroviral Therapy clinical trial. Am J Public Health. 2010;100:1896-903.
28. Fichtenbaum CJ, Gerber JG, Rosenkranz SL, et al. Pharmacokinetic interactions between protease inhibitors and statins in HIV seronegative volunteers: ACTG Study A5047. AIDS. 2002;16:569-77.
29. Aslangul E, Assoumou L, Bittar R, et al. Rosuvastatin versus pravastatin in dyslipidemic HIV-1-infected patients receiving protease inhibitors: a randomized trial. AIDS. 2010;24:77-83.
30. Boccara F, Lang S, Meuleman C, et al. HIV and coronary heart disease: time for a better understanding. J Am Coll Cardiol. 2013;61:511-23.
31. Boccara F, Mary-Krause M, Teiger E, et al. Acute coronary syndrome in human immunodeficiency virus-infected patients: characteristics and 1 year prognosis. Eur Heart J. 2011;32:41-50.
32. D'Ascenzo F, Cerrato E, Biondi-Zoccai G, et al. Acute coronary syndromes in human immunodeficiency virus patients: a meta-analysis investigating adverse event rates and the role of antiretroviral therapy. Eur Heart J. 2012;33:875-80.
33. Lorgis L, Cottenet J, Molins G, et al. Outcomes After Acute Myocardial Infarction in HIV-Infected Patients: Analysis of Data From a French Nationwide Hospital Medical Information Database. Circulation. 2013;127:1767-74.
34. Ren X, Trilesskaya M, Kwan DM, et al. Comparison of Outcomes Using Bare Metal Versus Drug-Eluting Stents in Coronary Artery Disease Patients With and Without Human Immunodeficiency Virus Infection. Am J Cardiol. 2009;104:216-22.
35. Kakuda TN, Schöller-Gyüre M, Hoetelmans RM. Pharmacokinetic interactions between etravirine and non-antiretroviral drugs. Clin Pharmacokinet. 2011;50:25-39.
36. Daali Y, Ancrenaz V, Bosilkovska M, et al. Ritonavir inhibits the two main prasugrel bioactivation pathways in vitro: a potential drug-drug interaction in HIV patients. Metabolism. 2011;60:1584-9.
37. Zhou D, Andersson TB, Grimm SW. In vitro evaluation of potential drug-drug interactions with ticagrelor: cytochrome P450 reaction phenotyping, inhibition, induction, and differential kinetics. Drug Metab Dispos. 2011;39:703-10.

CHAPTER 11

Perioperative Myocardial Infarction

INTRODUCTION

Myocardial ischemia, often followed by myocardial infarction (MI) is a known and much feared complication of noncardiac surgery. This condition has an in-patient mortality of 5–17%.[1,2,3] Mortality due to perioperative myocardial infarction (PMI) is particularly high in the first 30 days after a noncardiac surgery and it is an independent risk factor for cardiovascular death.

The Vascular Events in Noncardiac Surgery Patients Cohort Evaluation (VISION) study in 2017 revealed that as many as 65–93% of the patients with PMI have no ischemic symptoms,[2,3] and 50% of the cases of PMI remain unrecognized.[4] It is not surprising that findings of these studies pose a diagnostic dilemma. It is known that for clinical purposes, MI is broadly classified as ST segment elevation myocardial infarction (STEMI) and non-ST segment elevation myocardial infarction (NSTEMI). However, the concept of myocardial injury after noncardiac surgery (MINS) is more useful and broader. MINS is defined as prognostically relevant myocardial injury due to ischemia that occurs within 30 days after a noncardiac surgery.[5] The definition of MINS was primarily introduced to focus on the prognostic relevance of a peak in the Roche fourth-generation Elecsys troponin T (TnT) assay. As per the definition, serum levels of cardiac TnT (cTnT) which is higher than 0.03 ng/mL secondary to myocardial ischemia within 30 days after noncardiac surgery is significant. MINS is independently associated with 30-day mortality after noncardiac surgery—especially in patients undergoing vascular surgery.[5] Since sepsis and/or pulmonary embolism are some of the noncardiac conditions where troponin levels are elevated, it is important to distinguish between MINS and other noncardiac causes of elevated troponin levels.

■ PATHOPHYSIOLOGY

Even though the precise pathophysiological mechanisms of PMI are not clearly understood, it is different from nonoperative MI. Plaque fissuring and plaque rupture or acute thrombosis of the lumen in the coronary arteries characterize the nonoperative MI. However, two distinct mechanisms are described in patients with PMI.

Firstly, increase in luminal shear stress, endothelial activation, or inflammatory process lead to plaque instability and rupture—leading to thromboembolic dynamic obstruction of the arterial lumen.[6,7] The following mechanisms are likely to result in embolic obstruction:
- Pain, anemia and hypothermia associated with noncardiac surgery trigger increased release of catecholamines and cortisol which in turn cause vasoconstriction and plaque instability
- Increased vascular shear stress caused by tachycardia and hypertension may result in rupture of vulnerable plaques
- Surgery-induced procoagulant and antifibrinolytic activity is thought to precipitate coronary thrombosis in patients with or without coronary artery disease (CAD). Perioperative period is known to increase procoagulant levels (fibrinogen and von Willebrand factor) and reduce the levels of anticoagulant factors (protein C, antithrombin III and alpha-2-macroglobulin)
- Surgical trauma is known to set off a cascade of inflammatory markers such as tumor necrosis factor (TNF)-α, interleukin (IL)-1, IL-6 and C-reactive proteins. These markers can trigger plaque fissuring, rupture and acute coronary thrombosis.[6-10]

The second proposed mechanism is the imbalance between myocardial oxygen demand and supply in patients with chronic CAD. This imbalance between oxygen supply and demand can be a result of the following factors:
- Increased sympathetic activity triggered by surgery or anesthesia
- Hypotension caused by hypovolemia, bleeding or anemia
- Tachycardia due to anesthesia and arterial hypertension during intubation, extubation and hypothermia
- In the setting of significant coronary artery stenosis, there can be perioperative hypoxia or hypercarbia as a result of respiratory depression.[11]

Typically, perioperative myocardial ischemia occurs early in the postoperative period (peak occurrence, 100 minutes after surgery). In one study, majority of the ischemic events (67%) started within 2 hours from the end of surgery and emergence from anesthesia.

If administered without any complications, anesthesia in and of itself, whether general or regional, is not a risk factor in high-risk cardiac patients undergoing noncardiac surgery. However, postoperative stress (including emergence from anesthesia) triggers ischemia, infarction or both.

Intraoperative myocardial ischemia is less common and it is infrequently associated with PMI. Imbalance between oxygen demand and supply which is responsible for most cases of PMI is more important. Pre-existing CAD is a strong predictor of PMI and related morbidity. Type 2 NSTEMI is more common than type 1 STEMI.[12]

■ DIAGNOSIS

Prompt and timely recognition of PMI is of paramount importance. The attending anesthetist must rely on clinical signs and technology for the diagnosis of PMI because most of these patients are asymptomatic. The classic complaint of chest pain is an unreliable symptom in a patient who is awake because of the presence of confounding variables in the perioperative period (e.g. use of pain medications). Devereaux et al. found in a pooled data from multiple studies that just over 14% of the patients experiencing PMI actually complained of chest pain.[11]

Persistent hypotension with possible nausea and diaphoresis is one of the frequently encountered initial findings in patients experiencing perioperative myocardial ischemia.[13] A dip in oxygen saturation and electrocardiogram (ECG) changes are some of the other reliable signs.

Hypotension

An analysis by Bijker et al. revealed that at least 64% of the patients under anesthesia experienced episodes of drop in systolic blood pressure which is lower than 90 mm Hg. This study also revealed that more than 93% of the patients had at least one episode of mean arterial pressure that was 20% below the baseline.[14] Such a drop in blood pressure often resulted in adverse outcomes in the elderly patients. However, the clinical relevance of short-term and long-term implications of intraoperative hypotension continues to be mired in controversy. Monk et al. found that 1-year mortality increased by a factor of 3.6% for each minute that systolic blood pressure remained below 80 mm Hg.[15] Lienhart et al. conducted a review of perioperative deaths. This review found that intraoperative hypotension and anemia were closely associated with postoperative myocardial ischemic events.[13,16]

Electrocardiographic Changes

A standard 12-lead ECG is of great value and must be obtained. A ST segment depression and new T-wave inversion are the characteristic ECG changes in PMI. The ST segment changes can be seen well in leads V3–5, II and aVF. A ST-wave elevation (>1 mm) reflects subendocardial or transmural ischemia. The American College of Cardiology (ACC) defines the following ECG changes as meeting the criteria for PMI:
- New Q-wave changes (≥30 ms) present in any two contiguous leads fulfill the definition of the development of pathologic Q waves

- ECG changes indicative of ischemia are ST segment elevation (≥2 mm in lead V1, V2 or V3 and ST segment depression (≥1 mm) in at least two contiguous leads, or symmetric inversion of T waves (≥1 mm) in at least two contiguous leads.

The majority of the PMI are of the non-Q-wave type, preceded by episodes of ST segment depression and T-wave inversion.[12]

Postoperative ECG changes associated with troponin leak are independent predictors of mortality.[17] In the VISION study, postoperative ECG changes that were independently associated with 30-day mortality in the presence of elevated troponin levels included ST segment changes, left bundle branch block (LBBB), and ischemic changes in anterior leads.

Biomarkers

The myocardial tissue specificity of troponin biomarkers is almost absolute (100%). As little as 4-6% troponin leaks are associated with nonspecific cytosolic leaks. Elevated TnT levels should be evaluated by repeating the measurements at 3 hours and 6 hours including a delta between these time points. This helps to determine whether the elevation is acute or chronic.

Transesophageal Echocardiography

A study by Smith et al. was a landmark. This study provided almost unequivocal evidence that segment wall motion abnormalities detected through transesophageal echocardiography (TEE) are sensitive as well as specific indicators of myocardial ischemia.[18]

Angiography

Once the diagnosis of PMI is established through biomarkers and TEE, it is recommended that all patients should undergo coronary angiography (CAG) as early as feasible. This helps diagnose the cause of ischemia and guides further management. In the setting of NSTEMI, angiography is valuable in distinguishing between type 1 NSTEMI (plaque rupture or thrombosis) and type 2 NSTEMI (supply-demand imbalance). Invasive intervention is required to treat STEMI and type 1 NSTEMI. This can be determined only through prompt angiography.

■ MANAGEMENT OF PERIOPERATIVE MYOCARDIAL INFARCTION

Following are the most important goals in management of PMI:
- To confirm and validate the diagnosis of PMI by means of ECG and biomarker assays. It is irrespective of imaging
- Relief of myocardial ischemia
- To assess the hemodynamic status and correct the abnormalities if present
- Initiation of reperfusion.

Critical actions in the intraoperative period include the following:
- The surgery team and operating room (OR) staff must be immediately informed that patient's status might be compromised
- Adequate oxygenation must be ensured. The fraction of inspired oxygen (FiO_2) must be increased to 100%
- Depth of anesthesia should be decreased
- Monitoring must be expanded to include 12-lead ECG
- Fluid challenge should be initiated and a routine dose of phenylephrine should be given for the temporary management of the hypotension
- Hemodynamic stability must be quickly assessed. Other major acute causes of cardiovascular compromise must be ruled out. The other major causes include—hypovolemia, concealed hemorrhage, anaphylaxis, septic or neurogenic shock, anesthesia overdose, local anesthetic toxicity and tension pneumothorax
- Supportive measures to maintain blood pressure should be initiated. Vasopressin or epinephrine must be given to maintain coronary perfusion pressure (CPP) and cerebral perfusion pressure
- Arrhythmias, if any, must be corrected either pharmacologically or electrically or both. Amiodarone 150–300 mg bolus should be given for ventricular or atrial arrhythmias followed by subsequent infusion as needed. Synchronized cardioversion or defibrillation as indicated should be given. Epinephrine 1 mg q3–5 minutes for asystole as per Advanced Cardiac Life Support (ACLS) guidelines should be given
- In case of a cardiac arrest, standard cardiopulmonary resuscitation (CPR) must be carried out as per the ACLS guidelines
- Minimize myocardial work and oxygen demand while ensuring supply. Adequate oxygenation and ventilation should be ensured. Lower the heart rare with beta-blockers. Transfuse blood products to replace hemoglobin for improved delivery of oxygen. Avoid hypothermia and correct acidosis or other metabolic derangements
- Nitroglycerin must be administered to decrease preload while also dilating the coronary arteries
- Aspirin or another antiplatelet agent should be given if possible
- The laboratory tests such as arterial blood gas, electrolytes, basic metabolic panel (BMP) and complete blood count (CBC)
- Immediate order should be given for cardiac biomarker assay (cTnT or 5th-generation hsTnT)
- The ACC/AHA guideline for surveillance for troponin should be considered
- A central access must be immediately established if not done already. If present, its patency should be confirmed to permit large volume supportive resuscitation with fluids or blood products and inotropic infusions with vasopressors, if indicated
- Use of invasive monitoring must be considered, if not done already. Initiate arterial line-based, real-time, continuous cardiac output (CO)

and stroke volume variation (SVV) cardiac monitoring (e.g. with FloTrac or Vigileo) should be done. If a pulmonary catheter is already in place, assess CI and systemic vascular resistance (SVR). Look for pulmonary diastolic pressures and prominent A and V waves suggesting papillary muscle dysfunction and acute mitral regurgitation (MR). Use TEE to evaluate systolic and diastolic function, preload and afterload and valvular function—especially for evidence of new MR
- An intra-aortic balloon pump (IABP) for hemodynamic stability must be considered if a large anterior wall MI is diagnosed
- Consider extracorporeal membrane oxygenation (ECMO)
- Cardiology department must be notified for further management keeping in mind the possibility of an emergency need for coronary reperfusion therapy. A few randomized studies have been specifically directed at PMI and its outcomes. In majority of the times, guidelines for treatment of spontaneous acute coronary syndrome (ACS) are used while paying special consideration to the perioperative setting. Since thrombolytic therapy is contraindicated in STEMI, for the risk of bleeding, primary angioplasty in a cardiac catheterization laboratory is indicated
- Guidelines directed medical management of PMI should be considered in patients who have asymptomatic NSTEMI, for whom invasive reperfusion is not indicated or those with isolated elevation of cardiac biomarkers (i.e. MINS). Medical management of PMI must be done in collaboration with surgery team and cardiology as is the case during intraoperative management. Postoperative medical management of blood pressure, heart rate and pain should be aggressive to minimize stress and correct supply-demand imbalance.

REFERENCES

1. Devereaux PJ, Sessler DI. Cardiac complications in patients undergoing major noncardiac surgery. N Engl J Med. 2015;373(23):2258-69.
2. Devereaux PJ, Yang H, Yusuf S, et al. Effects of extended-release metoprolol succinate in patients undergoing non-cardiac surgery (POISE trial): a randomised controlled trial. Lancet. 2008;371(9627):1839-47.
3. Devereaux PJ, Biccard BM, Sigamani A, et al. Association of postoperative high-sensitivity troponin levels with myocardial injury and 30-day mortality among patients undergoing noncardiac surgery. JAMA. 2017;317(16):1642-51.
4. Devereaux PJ, Goldman L, Yusuf S, et al. Surveillance and prevention of major perioperative ischemic cardiac events in patients undergoing noncardiac surgery: a review. CMAJ. 2005;173(7):779-88.
5. Botto F, Alonso-Coello P, Chan MT, et al. Myocardial injury after noncardiac surgery: a large, international, prospective cohort study establishing diagnostic criteria, characteristics, predictors, and 30-day outcomes. Anesthesiology. 2014;120(3):564-78.
6. Bartels K, Karhausen J, Clambey ET, et al. Perioperative organ injury. Anesthesiology. 2013;119(6):1474-89.
7. Priebe HJ. Perioperative myocardial infarction—aetiology and prevention. Br J Anaesth. 2005;95(1):3-19.

8. Landesberg G, Beattie WS, Mosseri M, et al. Perioperative myocardial infarction. Circulation. 2009;119(22):2936-44.
9. Landesberg G. The pathophysiology of perioperative myocardial infarction: facts and perspectives. J Cardiothorac Vasc Anesth. 2003;17(1):90-100.
10. Devereaux PJ, Xavier D, Pogue J, et al. Characteristics and short-term prognosis of perioperative myocardial infarction in patients undergoing noncardiac surgery: a cohort study. Ann Intern Med. 2011;154(8):523-8.
11. Devereaux PJ, Goldman L, Cook DJ, et al. Perioperative cardiac events in patients undergoing noncardiac surgery: a review of the magnitude of the problem, the pathophysiology of the events and methods to estimate and communicate risk. CMAJ. 2005;173(6):627-34.
12. Landesberg G, Mosseri M, Zahger D, et al. Myocardial infarction after vascular surgery: the role of prolonged stress-induced, ST depression-type ischemia. J Am Coll Cardiol. 2001;37(7):1839-45.
13. Singh A, Antognini JF. Perioperative hypotension and myocardial ischemia: diagnostic and therapeutic approaches. Ann Card Anaesth. 2011;14(2):127-32.
14. Bijker JB, van Klei WA, Vergouwe Y, et al. Intraoperative hypotension and 1-year mortality after noncardiac surgery. Anesthesiology. 2009;111(6):1217-26.
15. Monk TG, Saini V, Weldon BC, et al. Anesthetic management and one-year mortality after noncardiac surgery. Anesth Analg. 2005;100(1):4-10.
16. Lienhart A, Auroy Y, Péquignot F, et al. Survey of anesthesia-related mortality in France. Anesthesiology. 2006;105(6):1087-97.
17. Biccard BM. Detection and management of perioperative myocardial ischemia. Curr Opin Anaesthesiol. 2014;27(3):336-43.
18. Smith JS, Cahalan MK, Benefiel DJ, et al. Intraoperative detection of myocardial ischemia in high-risk patients: electrocardiography versus two-dimensional transesophageal echocardiography. Circulation. 1985;72(5):1015-21.

INDEX

A

Abciximab administration, safety of 19
Activated clotting time 52
Activated partial thromboplastin time 20
Acute antiplatelet treatment 53
Acute coronary syndrome 2, 3, 9, 11, 29, 49, 52, 58, 60, 68, 72, 81-83, 85, 90, 91, 105, 116, 127
  treatment of 111
Acute myocardial infarction 1, 7, 16, 36, 59, 76, 82, 84, 86
  diagnosis of 60
  management of 60
Adenosine diphosphate 18
Advanced cardiac life support guidelines 126
AIDS 2
Alberta Kidney Disease Network 32, 33
Alteplase 12
American Association for Study of Liver Diseases 77
American College of Cardiology 30, 92, 124
American Heart Association 10, 30, 92
American Stroke Association 10
Anemia 123, 124
  autoimmune hemolytic 84, 85
Anesthesia 123
Angina, treatment of 111
Angiography 125
  coronary 18, 36, 82, 125
Angioplasty
  coronary 61
  primary 16
  stroke after primary 16
Angiotensin-converting enzyme 61
  inhibitor 4, 34, 63
  therapy 40
Antibody reaction 82
Anticoagulation 20
  agents 18
  periprocedural 52
  therapy 18
Antiphospholipid
  antibodies 83
  syndrome, primary 112
Antiplatelet 64
  therapy 18, 35
    timing of resumption of 21
  treatment 20, 75
Antiretroviral therapy 117
  management of 117
Antirheumatic drugs, disease-modifying 109
Antithrombotic therapy 40
Anxiety 97
Aorta, ascending 22
Aortic valve
  replacement 101
  stenosis 101
    symptomatic 101
Arrhythmias, cardiac 9
Arterial blood gas 126
Arterial disease, peripheral 30, 72
Aspirin 4, 20, 62
  low-dose 108, 109
  prophylactic use of 107
Atelectasis 97
Atherogenic lipid profile 116
Atherosclerosis 22, 30
  accelerated 108
  premature 108

B

Bare-metal stent 55
Beta-blockers 62, 76
Bivalirudin 52
Bleeding 123
  risk 53
Blood pressure 107, 118
  control of 34, 109
Body mass index 70
Bone mineral metabolism, disorders of 33

Brain 43
  tissue 14
Breast cancer 99
British National Lymphoma
  Investigation Database 86

C

Calcium channel antagonists 34
Cancer 90, 94, 95
Cardiac disease 90, 95, 108
Cardiocerebral infarction 8, 9
  hyperacute simultaneous 10
  synchronous 8
Cardiopulmonary bypass 75
Cardiovascular disease 1, 30, 101, 105, 116
  risk 117
Cardiovascular morbidity 106
Carotid artery
  stenosis 22
  stenting 23
Carotid endarterectomy 23
Carotid intima-media thickness 71
Carotid stenosis 22
  symptomatic 22
Carotid stenting 23
Cerebral artery
  anterior 14
  middle 11, 14
Cerebrovascular disease 1, 4
Charlson comorbidity index 1
Chemotherapy 98
  drugs 91
Child-Turcotte-Pugh classification 74
Cholesterol plaque formation 91
Chronic obstructive pulmonary disease 1, 58, 59, 61, 63, 64
Cigarette smoking, cessation of 118
Cirrhosis 71, 76
Clopidogrel 19, 53-55, 95
  plus aspirin 54, 55
Colon carcinoma 96
Combined combination antiretroviral therapy 116
Complete blood count 126
Connective tissue disease 1, 105
Conventional therapy 119
Coronary artery
  bypass grafting 42, 51, 61, 93, 96, 119
    surgery 18, 22, 23, 74
  calcification score 31
  disease 9, 30, 53, 59, 64, 69, 71, 72, 76, 82, 105, 108, 116, 123
    management of 119
    mechanisms of 91
    risk of 118
    stenosis, distribution of 70
    thrombosis 85
Coronary computed tomography angiography 69, 70
Coronary flow velocity reserve 31
Coronary heart disease 32
  atherosclerotic 85
  treatment of 35
Coronary perfusion pressure 126
Coronary reperfusion strategies 38
Coronary revascularization 61
Corticosteroids 113
Creatine kinase, isoenzymes of 43
Cyclooxygenase-2 selective inhibitors 108

D

Dabigatran 54, 55
Danazol 82
Deep vein thrombosis 12, 20
Dementia 1
Dermatomyositis 113
Diabetes 30, 33, 116
  mellitus 2, 71
Digestive tract tumors 95
Digital subtraction angiogram 15
Direct oral anticoagulant 53, 55
Disseminated intravascular coagulation 74
Dobutamine stress echocardiography 77
Drug-eluting stent 55, 93, 119
Dual antiplatelet therapy 22, 54, 73
Dyslipidemia 30, 33, 116, 118

E

Echocardiography, transesophageal 125
Emboli, chemical composition of 14
Endothelial dysfunction 30
Endothelial surface 83
Enzymes, cardiac 9
Epicardial adipose tissue 31
Esophageal varices 74
Estimated glomerular filtration rate 29
Exercise 109

S

Sickle cell
 anemia 85
 disease 85
Sickness, dominant cause of 1
Single antiplatelet therapy 54, 55
Sjögren's syndrome 112
Solid tumor 2
Splenectomy 82
Spontaneous bacterial peritonitis prophylaxis 74
Stable angina, pharmacological treatment of 42
Standard medical therapy 39
Statins 41, 63, 106
 therapy 34
Steatohepatitis, nonalcoholic 72
ST-elevation myocardial infarction 8, 12, 37, 42, 83
Stenosis
 bilateral asymptomatic 22
 unilateral asymptomatic 22
Steroids 82
Streptokinase 12
Stress 97
Stroke 13, 19, 22, 53
 acute 15
 ischemic 7, 12
 hemorrhagic 15
 ischemic 9, 10
 symptoms of 14
 volume variation 127
ST-segment elevation myocardial infarction 4, 30, 60, 61, 122

Systemic lupus erythematosus 105, 107
Systemic vasculitis, primary 112

T

Tachycardia 123
Takayasu's arteritis 112
Takotsubo cardiomyopathy 92
Tenecteplase 12
Thrombocythemia, essential 84
Thrombocytopenia 82, 94
Thrombotic thrombocytopenic purpura 82
Ticagrelor 19
Tissue plasminogen activator 14
Transient ischemic attacks 9
Transjugular intrahepatic portosystemic shunts 74
Triglycerides 119
Tumor necrosis factor 30, 123

U

Unstable angina, pharmacological treatment of 42

V

Vascular disease, peripheral 1
Vasculitis, systemic 105
Vitamin K antagonist 55
von Willebrand disease 83
von Willebrand factor 40, 83

W

WOEST trial 53